TEACHING AND LEARNING ANAESTHESIA IN A MUSEUM

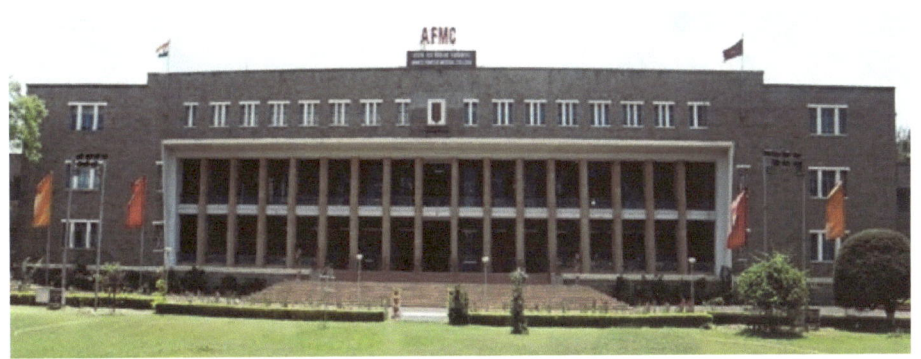

DR (COL) A K BHARGAVA

Ex Professor & Head
(Anaesthesiology and Critical Care)
Armed Forces Medical College
Pune

Former Director (Anaesthesiology)
Rajiv Gandhi Cancer Institute & Research Centre
New Delhi

The mission of creating an Anaesthesia Museum should be to 'Advance Anesthesiology by Preserving and Sharing its Heritage and Knowledge'. This is what the changing faculty of Anesthesiology at Armed Forces Medical College is sincerely pursuing.

CONTENTS

FOREWORD-1	7
FOREWORD-2	8
PREFACE	9
INTRODUCTION	10
HISTORY	12
ANATOMY	16
OXYGEN THERAPY AND RESUSCITATION	41
ENDOTRACHEAL ANAESTHESIA	52
REGIONAL ANAESTHESIA	63
DRUGS CONCERNING ANAESTHESIOLOGISTS	66
ANAESTHETIC ANCILLARIES	70
MONITORING & MONITORING EQUIPMENT	73
CARDIAC ANAESTHESIA	82
CRITICAL CARE	85
CONCLUSION	87
REFERENCES	88

FOREWORD-1

FOREWORD

The process of teaching has many facets. Didactic lecturing is easy to organize but falls far short of the objectives when it has to deal with a patient oriented discipline like Anaesthesiology. Practical "apprenticeship" does afford hands-on experience but again does not afford an insight into the theoretical bases of various aspects of a technology-oriented speciality like Anaesthesia. The appliances and instruments of anaesthesia have undergone a sea change from the times of Snow and Morton. As in all the fields of science there has been an exponential increase in the degree of sophistication to the extent that one tends to believe that the principles have changed. In fact, the situation is somewhat like the plight of the biologist looking at a human being and a fish and trying to link the two. What my enthusiastic colleague Dr. Bhargava has done is rather like the approach of a biologist. He has collected all the old appliances (that have lived their useful life) and linked them up to weave a 'fossil' story in Anaesthesiology. What an interesting use of teaching material that would have been junked. I have sauntered through this museum and come out quite enlightened. I am sure this novel approach is effective and that this compilation will be well received. I would urge the readers to pay a visit to the original museum in the Armed Forces Medical College that has been painstakingly built up by successive members of the faculty of the anaesthesiology department.

24 Jan 1994

Maj Gen D Raghunath
Dean & Dy Commandant
AFMC; Pune

FOREWORD-2

Foreward

Foundations of Anaesthesiology were laid in the 19th century and systematization of the art was accomplished in the 20th century. The anaesthesia museum at AFMC can boast to have one of largest collection of exhibits pertaining to latter half of the 19th and early half of the 20th century. It is interesting to note that several pieces of apparatuses that are now obsolete, not only illustrate a particular feature but also are periodically re-invented. Hence, the need for preservation of antique equipment, for the purpose of study in a particular field.

The museum got a face lift after the Anaesthesiology Department shifted from the dilapidated II World War barracks to the newly raised Golden Jubilee Block of AFMC in 1998. The development of the museum is largely due to our enthusiastic colleague Col AK Bhargava who has been instrumental in its organization and who is also the author of this very well illustrated monograph which will not only serve as a guide for visitors to the museum but also infuse enthusiasm within the postgraduates and students of the graduate wing.

An effort is being initiated to launch a website of the museum and link it with that of the Armed Forces Medical College. The evolution of Anaesthesia can be appreciated by visiting the museum and I would like to invite teachers and students of other institutions to visit this museum which is probably the only one of its type in Asia and the rare ones across the globe.

I would like to compliment Col AK Bhargava, Professor of the Department of Anaesthesiology & Critical Care and acknowledge his excellent efforts towards this novel project.

Date: 19 Aug 2003

Lt Gen VD Tiwari
Director & Commandant
AFMC, Pune

PREFACE

PREFACE

When planning and considering the various methods of education one considers whether a lecture, group discussion, slide presentation, a chalk board or computer assisted instructional software is better than the other but little is thought of the role of a museum on this aspect

A museum is an institution for collection preservation and display of objects of interest. An Anaesthesia museum may sound strange to some and of little logic to others. Though not listed in any of the directory of any museum, the Anaesthesia museum at the Armed Forces Medical College, Pune; developed its foundations with the establishment of the college in 1962. The uniqueness of this museum lies in the fact that it is probably the only type of its kind in the world in a medical college which itself is a unique institution run by the Armed Forces of a country. That the museum is peculiar is further established by the fact that there is no director, curator, conservator or registrar; it is only the changing faculty that has been contributing a wee bit each time during the tenure at the college. It was only during the last few years that an attempt and concerted effort at reorganization and update was conducted to convert this museum from a storehouse to a place of teaching and learning.

An update of this monograph is now reconducted during my second tenure at the college, and hope it will now give a broader outlook to the students and residents

Col AK Bhargava
Professor and Head
Dept of Anaesthesiology
Armed Forces Medical College

INTRODUCTION

A systematic survey of all apparatuses and devices that exist in the inventory of the Department of Anaesthesiology at Armed forces Medical College since its inception had been rearranged and numerous unwanted items removed together with addition of text and literature in order to make one interested in the subject. The aim of addition of such matter has been to give a broader outlook to the residents in Anaesthesiology on the subject. It is also aimed to give an insight to the medical graduates the role an Anaesthesiologist plays in the medical profession and to make them interested in a subject which is less discussed at the undergraduate level. The Department of Anaesthesiology at the Armed Forces Medical College was located in a II World War barrack with a room containing junked equipment. In 1995 it found its way on the top floor of the Golden Jubilee Block. The Department of Anaesthesiology & Critical Care can now boast to be one of the finest departments of the institution. It was here that the idea of creation of a museum for teaching and learning was thought of. An attempt was made to define certain sections in the museum to keep the house in order. Starting with history, followed by anaesthetic apparatuses, oxygen therapy and resuscitation, endotracheal anaesthesia, regional anaesthesia, drugs used in anaesthesia, cardiac anaesthesia, monitoring and lastly critical care were incorporated.

A modest beginning had been initiated and web pages were created in the AFMC website concerning the museum. After scanning through the web pages of AFMC, many Anaesthesiologists may be tempted to visit the museum and Armed Forces Medical College would be too happy to welcome them. Being a medical graduate from the same institution I never remember having visited the Anaesthesia Department but as a teacher in the same Department, I am convinced of the fact that the museum is an important media by which we can convey the message which we think is essential to the undergraduates. The object of this exercise is not to try collecting and compiling all that exists pertaining to Anaesthesia but to make a comprehensive account in systematic manner of the inventory which exists on ground.

HISTORY

History is of practical value to the Anaesthetist. The value of history is that it enables us to avoid making too often the mistakes that others have already made. Many a time repetitions have been committed because of our ignorance of what is happening around us. Hence it is a must that we ought to know what our forefathers did. Many items described may seem too stupid and dangerous whereas others highly ingenious. The Department of Anaesthesiology and Critical Care was earlier located in the barrack accommodation of the British Army and was later housed on the top floor of the Golden Jubilee Block.

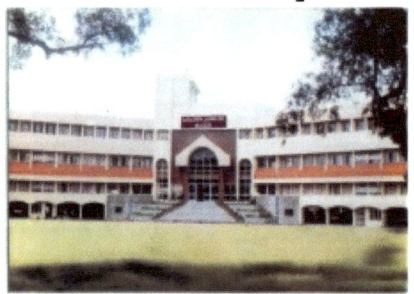 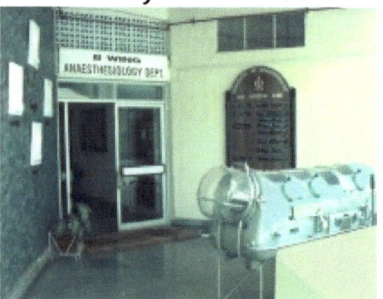

It is from the entrance to the Department itself that the museum begins. Four eminent personalities and amongst the greatest pioneers in Anaesthesiology and the iron lung adorn the entrance.

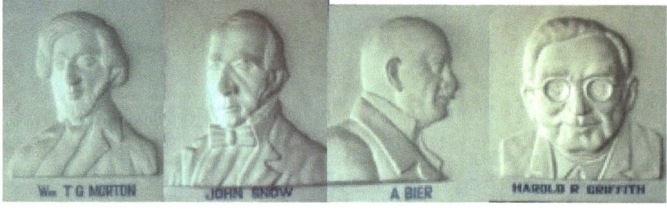

William Thomas Green Morton (1819-1868), John Snow (1813-1858), A Bier (1861-1949) and Harold R Griffith (1894-1985) remind every student entering the department to pay tributes to these epoch makers.

Morton and Snow will always find a place in any textbook in Anaesthesiology. Their contribution on the design of various inhalers for ether and chloroform was the beginning of an era on vaporization and vaporizers. The tabloid on **Morton** grave states "Inventor and revealer of inhalational anaesthesia before whom in all time, surgery was agony; by whom, pain in surgery was averted and annulled; since whom, science had control over pain".

'Anaesthesia Day' is celebrated on 16th October in many parts of the globe as on this day Morton demonstrated the first successful anaesthetic in man in 1846.

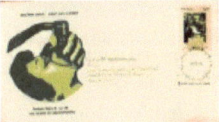

The Govt of India has also recognized this achievement by issuing a **First day cover** by the Post & Telegraphs Dept in 1997. 150 yrs. after this historic event, **John Snow** was the first full time anaesthetist during the middle of the last century and had the honour of administering chloroform to Queen Victoria on the births of Prince Leopold and Princess Beatrice in an attempt to provide pain relief in labour. He was responsible for converting Anaesthesia from art to science. A **Bier** is known as the "Initiator" of spinal analgesia and **Griffith** is known for the "Introducer" of muscle relaxants. The 'Iron Lung', one of the massive exhibits which could not be housed within the museum room, had to be left outside as a showpiece and ornamental value at the entrance of the Department. It is discussed under the heading of resuscitation.

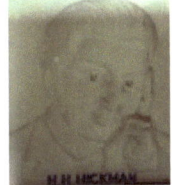 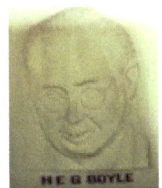 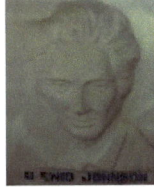

Other personalities **HH Hickman, HEG Boyle and Enid Johnson** - whose figures in clay were also prepared in the early years of the college, can be seen in the museum. Hickman was able to perform surgical operations painlessly on animals in 1824 by causing them to inhale carbon dioxide. His was the first work on surgical anaesthesia by inhaling a gas. Boyle in 1917 got Coxeter the instrument maker to copy Gwathmeys gas-oxygen machine that became the first 'Boyles apparatus'. He introduced gas oxygen into France for use in anaesthetising soldiers in World War I and for this he received the decoration of the OBE. Johnson with Griffith used curare for the first time to relaxation during surgery in 1942 in Montreal. Dates are important in any history. A chart depicting the important events the world over is displayed. India had its contributions in the enhancement of the specialty.

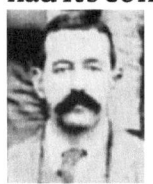

Surgeon-Major Edward Lawrie of Hyderabad was a great protagonist of chloroform and had taken active part in initiating the Hyderabad commissions to counter the adverse effects of chloroform and prove the then currently prevailing Edinburgh school of thought (that respiration and not circulation should be watched) to be correct. The two Hyderabad commissions on chloroform (1888 and 1889) appeared to have started and concluded without an unbiased scientific observation. It ought to be recalled that it was concluded in these commissions that chloroform is never a primary cardiac depressant. This is now known to be untrue. The establishment of Indian Society of Anaesthetists in 1947 is important dates for Indian history. The idea to form an All India Society was originated during the centenary celebration of ether anaesthesia held in Bombay in 1946 and the first All India conference of the Indian Society of Anaesthetists (ISA) was held on 24/25th Dec 1949. A copy of the Constitution of ISA is displayed in this section. The Society published its first journal in July 1953. A Memorabilia was published by ISA in 1997 on its 50th birth anniversary. A copy of the same is displayed. The Pune city branch of Anaesthesiology which is affiliated to the ISA was formed in

1970.Subsequently other societies (research society of Anaesthesiology & Clinical Pharmacology, Critical Care Society) under various banners have formed. The fact that Anaesthesiology has become a popular specialty is forthcoming by the fact that as of today there are now as many as 15 state and 66 city branches of the Indian Society of Anaesthesiologists, it must be recalled that in 1941-42 leading anaesthetists from Great Britain arrived in India for service in the Armed Forces. Some of the names from the records are Dr H.K.Asheworth, Dr T.A.B.Harris, Dr U.F.Hall and Dr W.S.McConnel.

Anesthesiology as a subject has now become a major specialty in medicine with many subspecialties emerging on the horizon. With the importance of the subject The Department got a boost in 2010 when it was finally given space in the main building of Armed Forces Medical College (see cover).

ANATOMY

Ellis, the author of 'Anatomy for anaesthetists', would have been greatly pleased to see a section of anatomy in this museum. A full size female **human skeleton** gives a welcome to this section. Some amount of Osteology ought not to be forgotten by practicing anaesthesiologists for reasons to be mentioned.

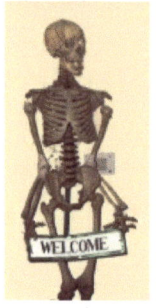

A cut human skull giving details of the base of the skull, the various vertebrae, ribs, clavicle and pelvis are at display separately. Understanding regional anaesthesia and acupuncture requires an in-depth study of the skeletal system and applied anatomy. Somehow the science of Acupuncture interested many Anaesthesiologists because of the remarkable relief of pain in many illnesses. Again, the triad of Anaesthesia (Hypnosis, Analgesia and Muscle relaxation) could be achieved by performing acupuncture and acupuncture anaesthesia took shape. Life size **Acupuncture models**, male and female depicting the meridians and points had been procured in the dept in the early 80's.

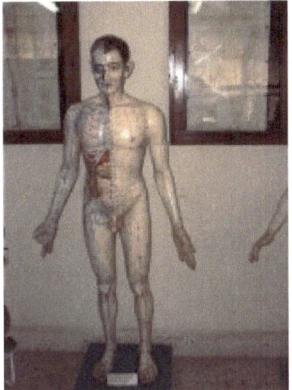
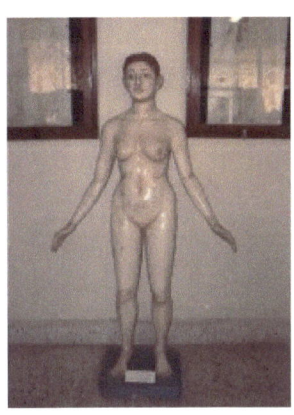
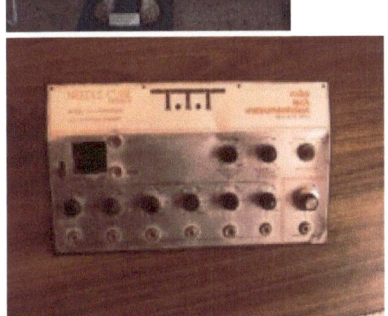

Acupuncture equipment (Battery operated acupuncture stimulators and point locators) of that period are also displayed. This section is therefore appropriately placed diametrically opposite the Regional Anaesthesia section for the purpose of learning. Models and charts on the larynx, pharynx, bronchopulmonary segments and heart are shown in detail; conveying the importance of the cardiopulmonary system to any anaesthesiologist. It may be recalled that as early as the latter part of the nineteenth century it was taught to any practicing anaesthetist to watch the pulse while giving chloroform and respiration while giving ether. During my days in the 1st professional of MBBS, I had hardly imagined I would be peering through so many larynxes' in my career to follow. At that time, I had hardly understood the intricacies of the larynx and I wonder why in the Anatomy Department in the same institution did not have models of a **mechanical larynx** similar to the one in the museum.

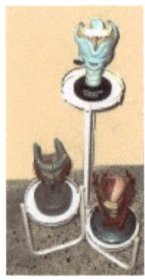

 Physiology is probably a more useful subject in anaesthesiology because under anaesthesia we tend to keep all physiological parameters within normal limits. A preanaesthetic evaluation is therefore a must for the safe conduct of anaesthesia.

ANAESTHETIC APPARATUS

Devices for administering inhalational volatile anaesthetics have been an ongoing process. The early development of anaesthesia from 1846 to the beginning of First World War saw a number of ingeniously designed devices. During this period both ether and chloroform rivaled each other for superiority.

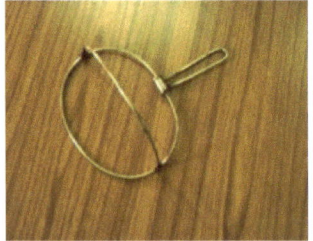

Many exhibits in the museum pertain to this era. Some of the devices cannot be ascribed to the originator but would never the less be discussed. The first and probably the oldest is the **Skinner's Inhaler**. Thos Skinner (1862) was an obstetrician in Liverpool who designed this domette covered wire framed mask which has since been imitated by others.

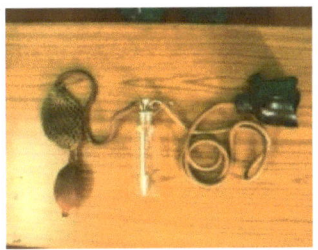

In 1867 **Junker's inhaler** was popular. This was introduced by F.E. Junker a German surgeon in London. It consists of (Hand bellows, a chloroform bottle and a face piece). Air is pumped through a certain depth of chloroform contained in a bottle, and the vapour conveyed to the patient by means of the face mask. Though an attempt was made in this inhaler to deliver a known percentage of the vapour it is in no way better than the open method of administration because the small quantity of high percentage vapour is diluted by a much larger quantity of air inspired from the general atmosphere. None the less it could be well considered the fore runner of the plenum vaporizers in the decades to follow.

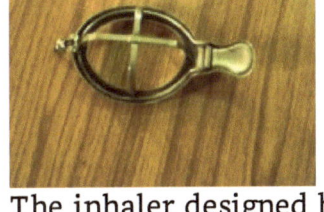

The inhaler designed by **Carl Schimmelbusch** of Berlin in 1890 had remained a popular device for both ether and chloroform and surprisingly in many of the third world countries it is still being used for the purpose of anaesthesia for the former agent.

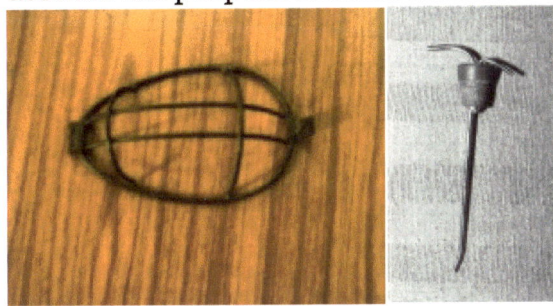

A similar wire frame device which more closely fits the face was that devised by **Bellamy Gardner** in 1907. An **ether dropper** which too was designed by him goes by his name. The dropper is a rubber stopper adapted for an ordinary six-ounce bottle; the long metal tube dips into the ether, the short one allows air to enter the bottle to replace the ether used. The present day ether bottles take this dropper easily; probably this is why the present manufacturers of ether have not changed their dispensing bottles.

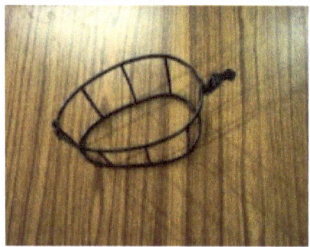

Ogston of Aberdeen around the same time designed a wire frame inhaler with several vertical struts, united at their distal end by a ring. Round these struts a towel was pinned. This frame could then be fixed on the wire frame similar to the Bellamy Gardner. This technique converted the system into a somewhat semi-open method which not only helped in attaining a higher concentration of ether with passage of time but was also economizing on the ether used.

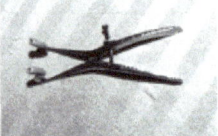

Mason had invented a mouth gag in 1871. A mouth gag inhaler which has combined features of the Masons gag with an extended wire frame is one of the exhibits which cannot be traced to its founder. It was probably a device to help in dental extraction or some form of oral surgery.

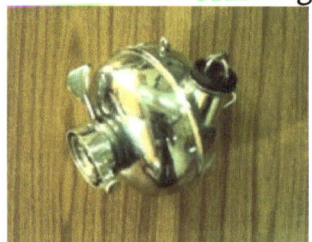

Hewitt in 1901 described his wide bore ether inhaler which worked on the same principle as Clover's inhaler but differed in having less resistance during inspiration (ingress) and expiration (egress) of air. The construction also differs in that to turn on the ether instead of rotating the drum the indicator is moved.

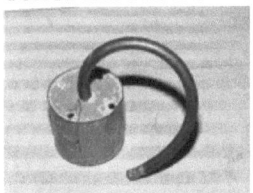

Flagg's Can an ingenuity of World War 1 (1919), and subsequently used by Macintosh and Pratt during the Spanish Civil War in 1939 and Thornton in World War II. This "tin can "with multiple perforations on its top is a simple ether inhaler to be used in conjunction with an endotracheal tube is still fancied in the underdeveloped world and refined versions of the same made of plastic, corrugated tubing's and one way valves are in production. Though N_2O was discovered by Colton in 1863 it found its use in clinical practice with the development of machines for delivery of the gas by the end of the nineteenth century. Simpler devices utilizing N_2O had been devised in the last century.

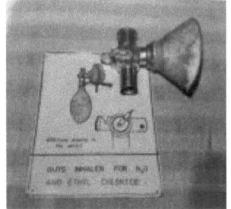

Guy's inhaler for the administration of N2O and Ethyl chloride induction unit dates as far back as 1870. It comprises of a three way stop cock whose horizontal limb is prolonged half an inch. In each side of the prolongation is a hole. The bag mount has in its side also one hole, which is connected by a universal ball and socket joint with the rubber tube, to which an ethyl chloride vial is attached. A pointer on the outside of the bag mount serves as an indicator to show that the ethyl chloride vial is in continuity with the interior of the inhaler. N_2O and O_2 can be introduced into the system by a tube in the bag mount. It must be realized however that the apparatus was used as a single dose method of administering N_2O and ethyl chloride.

Teter's was the earliest gas oxygen outfit that made possible the use of rebreathing, positive pressure and addition of ether vapour to the gases. Gwathmey introduced the sight feed type of flowmeters. Both Heidbrink and Boyles machines were descendants of the Teter's machine. J.Heidbrink(1913) in U.S.A and H.E.G. Boyle(1917) in Britain had attained a remarkable refinement of anaesthetic machines and formed the basis on which the present technology is based. In 1906 Franz Kuhn in Germany recognized the use of CO_2 absorbers in anaesthetic circuits.

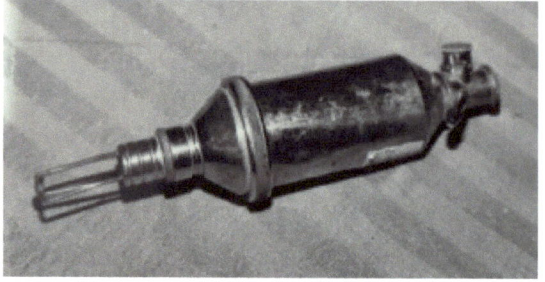 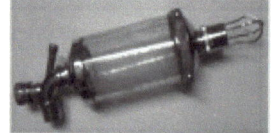

The **soda lime to and fro absorber** was first described by Ralph Waters in 1923. Even **paediatric to and fro absorbers** with a modified T piece were in practice. Brian Sword overcame the awkward position of the canister near the patients face by introducing the circle system in 1930. Thereafter all machines in Europe and America had provision of a circle system. At first the directional valves consisted of rubber flaps at the patient end of the hosing but subsequently the American innovation of gravity type valves incorporated in the body of the absorber was adopted and became standard practice.

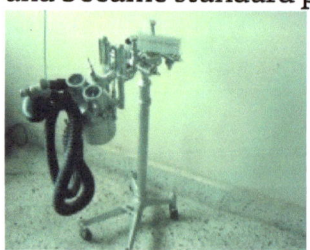

Heidbrinks portable anaesthetic apparatus had a circle type absorber with an ether vaporizer situated on the expiratory side of the circuit. A control is provided for inclusion and exclusion of the CO_2 absorber from the circuit. The purpose of the control in those days was to allow the concentration of CO2 to rise in the circuit. The unit incorporates the typical heidbrink flowmeters.

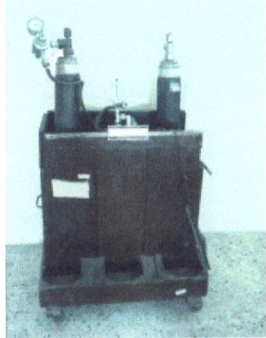

One of the **Earliest versions of the Boyles apparatus** after the World War 1 can be seen in the museum. It is designed on a wooden frame mounted on castors. It has a triple sight feed water-bubble flowmeter for delivering N2O, O2 and CO2 and measuring their rates of flow. Each of the tubes has five perforations at half inch intervals. There are chloroform and ether Bakelite mounted bottles and their outlet is supposed to be connected to a 2 gallon rubber bag with a **Barth 3 way** or similar stopcock and rubber padded face piece.

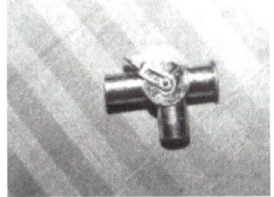

The **standard stopcocks** in those days had three positions. In "Air" position the patient breathes air only; the outlet of the bag being shut off. In the "Valves" position inspiration of patient draws gas from the bag and expiration is conducted to the atmosphere. In the "No Valves" position inhalation takes place from the bag and exhalation takes place into it. (Note: Guys inhaler incorporates in the apparatus a 3 way stop cock too). A metallic chain from the back bar upto the ground level is part of the machine. Knowledge of the danger of generation of electrostatic charge was possibly well recognized.

This machine was supposed to have **fine adjustment valves** fitted to the cylinders of the gases to permit even control of flow of gases. The gases were then fed by rubber tubing's to the water filled bubble type flowmeters. If by chance the control on the flowmeter is closed the connector rubber tube has a tendency to get blown off due to the high pressure build up.

Many devices those days had twin N2O cylinders (one for use and one for reserve) which were interconnected through a metal union with fly nuts. To allow N2O flow the assembly was opened with the help of a specially designed **Nitrous oxide cylinder key** on the disc on the metal union. The cylinders themselves were available in a wide range varying from number 25 to 3500. The size number indicating the volume (gallons) of gas which the fluid contents will give off at atmospheric pressure. In Britain they were painted black.

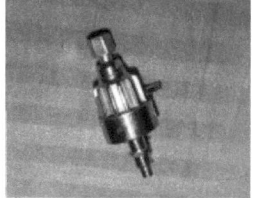

In 1923 **Adams** designed the **pressure reducing valve** which produced a reduced and regulated pressure of 5 lbs/sq". This enabled the fine control valves to be fitted on the flowmeters themselves without fear of having been blown off by any accumulating pressure. The dry flowmeter with fine control valves was designed by Coxeter and incorporated in the Boyles machine in 1933. Rotameters though patented as early as 1907 in Germany by Karl Kuppers, were used by Magill in 1932 and finally Salt in 1937 who perfected it to be incorporated in the Boyles machine in the same year. A further refinement in the machine was made around 1940 when Magill's rebreathing attachment comprising a bag mount with an on/off stop cock, one gallon bag, corrugated breathing tube, expiratory valve (Heidbrink pattern) and face piece substituted the Barth connection and the larger 2-3 gallon gas bag. This was in accordance with the concept of continuous flow principle of gas and O2 supply.

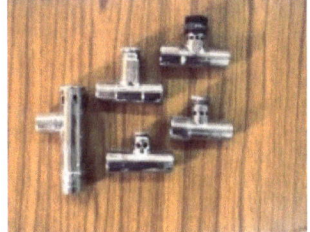

Various types of expiratory valves somewhat similar to the **Heidbrink, McKesson, Minnet and Salt valves** are displayed.

Face masks of rubber, bakelite, metal, with and without or incorporated inflatable pads have been manufactured from time to time. Some versions of these face pieces are on display.

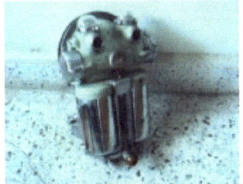

A new **circle type CO_2 absorber Coxeter-Mushin** was described by W.W.Mushin in 1943.

This design showed several new features: (a) although constructed on the two phase principle with uni-directional valves, both phases of respiration are directed through the soda lime canister; (b) the inbuilt ether chamber had baffles to enhance the vaporization; (c) a concertina-shaped re-breathing bag was fitted with a counter balanced control lever which reduces to a minimum the inertia that had to be overcome at the initiation of inspiration. The Boyle's machine although named after the anaesthetist who originated it, is actually a trade mark belonging to the British Oxygen Company.

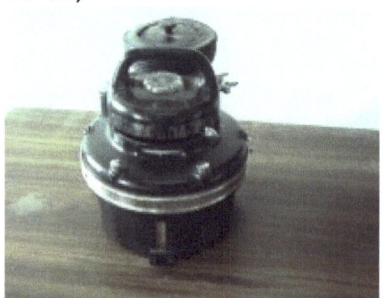

The **standard Boyles machine (Model G)** of the 40's was a metal table with castors, fitted with metal baskets to carry the gas cylinders. Atop the cylinders were fitted the Adam's valves and rubber tubing connected them to the rotameters. The bakelite mounted vaporizers had a plunger device. A Magill's rebreathing attachment was provided and the Coxeter-Mushin absorption unit was an optional unit. During the 2nd World War period in 1941,

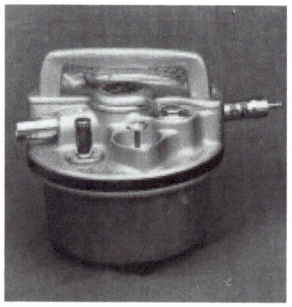

Dr HG Epstein, physicist in the Oxford Dept and Professor Macintosh of Oxford with Mendelssohn devised the **Oxford vaporizer** which was the forerunner of the famous **EMO inhaler.** The Oxford Vaporizer prepares ether vapour and this is inhaled in a concentration controlled by the anaesthetist. It is independent of gas and oxygen cylinders although a tap is provided for O_2 if desired. The vehicle for ether vapour is air which is drawn through the apparatus with each inspiration. In this apparatus ether is vaporized at constant temperature; the source of heat being the latent heat given off during the re-crystallization of $CaCl_2$ which has previously been fused by hot water poured into the central chamber. The process of fusion and re-crystallization of $CaCl_2$ can be continued indefinitely, the crystals being in a sealed chamber.

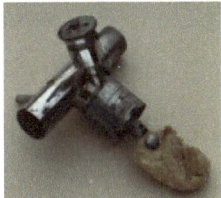

To make induction easier; a special **ethyl chloride induction unit** was designed so that it could be attached to the breathing circuit of the Oxford vaporizer.

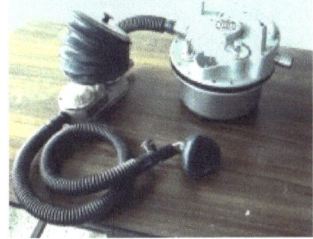

The **Draw over vaporising unit (EMO with OIB)** designed by Epstein and Macintosh at Oxford in 1952 was clearly the most popular draw over inhalational devices developed. In the Indian Armed Forces this apparatus had been the backbone of anaesthetic equipment in the far fletched remote areas of the country where the Army has been deployed. The OIB (Oxford Inflating Bellows) by themselves form a useful device for manual ventilation. The Heidbrink expiratory valve is provided with the patient circuit. In case a non-return valve is to be used then the unidirectional valve of the OIB towards the patient end is immobilized with the help of a magnet provided. Alternative scales were developed so that apart from ether it could be used for trichlorethylene and halothane.

Though anaesthesia in obstetric practice dates as far back April 7th 1853 when Victoria, Queen of Great Britain and Empress of India was administered chloroform by Snow in order to produce analgesia not anaesthesia - 'Chloroform a lareine', for the birth of Prince Leopold. After this episode Mr. Wakley editor of Lancet

went on to publish in the same journal that 'in no case could it be justifiable to administer chloroform in normal labour'. Despite this and the reluctance of the royal obstetricians John Snow was called upon to administer chloroform to Queen Victoria again for the birth of Princess Beatrice in 1857. Thus pain relief for labour in history started with the assent of the Queen. In the early 1930's there was a great demand for a satisfactory method for providing pain relief during childbirth. Various apparatuses utilizing N2O were developed since
methods for storing and delivering N2O had been devised.

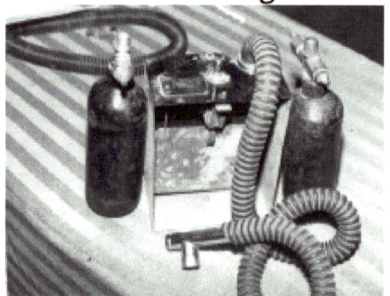 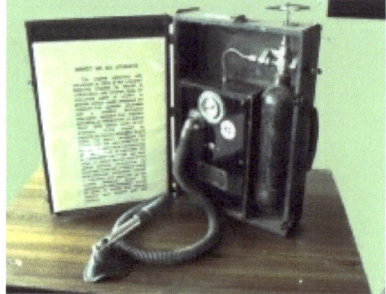

The **Walton-Minnet Air-Gas analgesia apparatus** developed in 1933 and the **Minnet Air-Gas analgesia apparatus** (Queen Charlotte model) of 1943 can be seen alongside.

In both apparatuses the main principle is that gas supply is controlled by a valve which only comes into operation during inspiration of the patient. The importance of both these machines lies in the fact that they were the forerunners of the intermittent flow anaesthetic machines to be designed in the second half of this century.

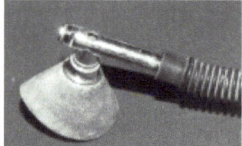

Interposed between the machine and patient after the corrugated tubing is an **expiratory valve** which also permits air via an aperture making it a 45% mixture of gas and air during the inspiratory phase.

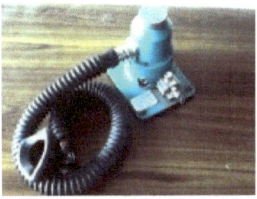

The **Cardiff inhaler** was designed in the 60's when methoxyflurane (Penthrane) was introduced and became very popular with midwives in UK. With the recognition of fluoride toxicity of penthrane the use of this device also declined.

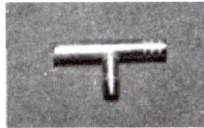

Phillip.T.Ayre of Newcastle in 1937 described the **"T" Piece** for administering endotracheal anaesthesia in infants and children. In his original documents Ayre stated the following advantages of the "T" piece. a) No obstruction to free respiration. b) No anoxaemia in case of oxygen exhaustion. c) Amount of rebreathing can be adjusted by altering the length of expiratory
limb by attaching a length of rubber tubing. d) Vascular congestion and haemorrhage are reduced
to a minimum.

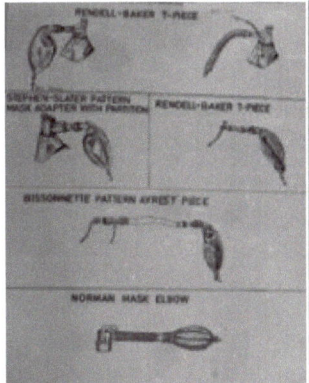 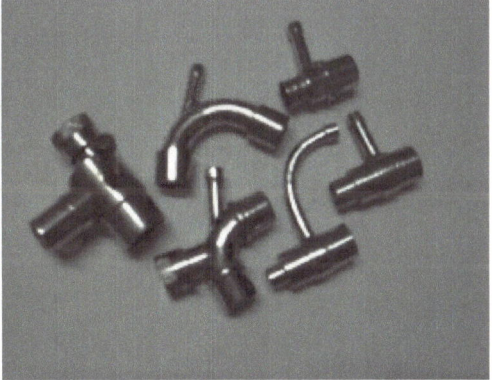

Ever since the "T" piece became popular various **Modified designs of the "T" piece** were produced eg. **Rendell Baker, Norman elbow, Cape Town, Nesi, Hustead, MIE, Khushwaqt**.
It was on the basis of the "T" piece that the subsequent semi closed circuits described by Rees (1950) and Mapleson (1954)

were described. Mapleson analysed five feasible ways, denoted from A-E in which a source of fresh gas, mask, reservoir bag, expiratory valve and length of wide bore tubing could be arranged to administer gases to a subject. Mapleson A system corresponds to the Magills circuit and has been advocated for spontaneous respiration whereas Mapleson D has been advocated for controlled ventilation. Willis (1975) added the F system to the original five arrangements. This is similar to the circuit described by Jackson Rees. The disadvantage of the A system is that the expiratory valve has limited accessibility and there is difficulty in scavenging. Many workers (Carden-1972, Lack-1975, Miller-1979, Voss-1985) modified this circuit to overcome these difficulties. The Lack coaxial version (outer tube with a diameter of 2.8cm, inner tube of 14mm diameter and length 1.5m) proved to be more popular than others though Voss's design of the "Enclosed Magill Anaesthetic Breathing system" proves to be efficient during controlled ventilation also. Bain and Spoerel (1972) described the Coaxial system which as we know today is in essence a modification of the D system. It comprises of an outer tube with a 22 mm internal diameter, inner tube with a 7 mm internal diameter and is 1.8 m long. Functionally the D, E, F, and Bain systems are similar. Combined systems (Waters-1961, Humphrey-1986) to incorporate the virtues of A system and D system have also been developed but in our country, they have not gained popularity. Another of the modifications of the Mapleson systems has been the removal of the valves altogether and in its place the gas is withdrawn at a rate equal to the fresh gas flow (Haffnia modification). In these systems the withdrawal is affected by an ejection flowmeter utilizing the venturi effect. The technique enables easier scavenging and offers less resistance. The British Oxygen Company (BOC) were the pioneers to manufacture and supply Anaesthetic machines and in independent India, Indian Oxygen Limited a subsidiary of BOC became the main suppliers. It was natural that American machines were hardly given any competition due to the British legacy. However, immediately after independence the Indian Army did procure anaesthesia machines which were of American origin.

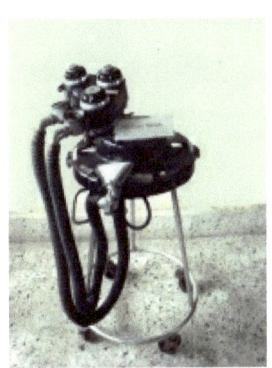 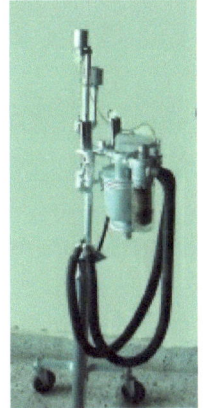

The **Merret machine** of Airmed and the **Ohio machine** of the Chemical & Surgical Equipment Co. manufactured in 1958 bear evidence to this. The Marret anaesthetic head is capable of being adjusted to give practically any closed or semi-closed breathing circuit. The trilene control includes a safety interlock. The Ohio machine incorporates within the breathing circuit a water manometer to measure the positive pressure in the breathing circuit. It too has facility for closed circuit circle system.

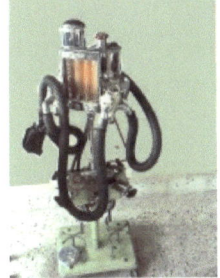

The **Gillis Machine** a British version of the modern machines of the early 1950's were being by practitioners in the civil. It is a portable machine with facilities for closed circuit anaesthesia.

This machine was being used by Dr Patwardhan in Pune till the turn of the century. After 50yrs of service to him he gifted this machine to the museum.

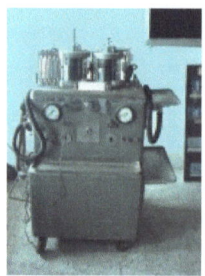

The **'Blease All Purpose Pulmoflator'** manufactured by Blease Anaesthetic Equipment Ltd. Ryefield crescent, Middlesex is truly one of sophistications reached in anaesthetic care. This is an impressive exhibit. Ventilator designs were developed in the 60's-70's to be used specifically during anaesthesia when muscle relaxants were introduced and the Liverpool technique of Balanced anaesthesia started becoming popular. The ventilator in this machine was designed for pressure and volume cycling, it has a variable inspiratory time and provision for inspiratory triggering. Both PEEP and Negative pressure during expiration could be employed. There was provision for inflating the arm band of the BP apparatus by the cylinder oxygen, suction apparatus working off the vacuum side of the rotary pump unit and an attachment for fitting bronchoscope whose light source came from a rheostat and transformer unit working inside the cabinet. Either semi closed or closed circuit could be employed and a provision for manual control was available.

IOL has manufactured various **Boyle's models** of anaesthesia machines in independent India. Most of them are illustrated in the various charts/posters displayed.

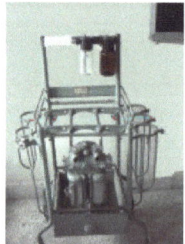

Model G as described earlier was the one having the Coxeter-Mushin absorption unit with cylinder baskets. Model H had the Boyle Mk 11 circle absorber instead of the Coxeter-Mushin one.

Cylinder baskets were eliminated and yoke assembly and hanger were used. Model E had the cyclopropane assembly removed.

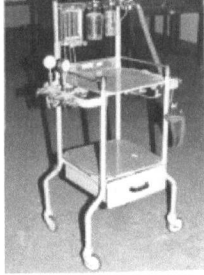

Model F was similar model E without any CO_2 absorber unit. Later models had the Adam's valves replaced with the preset regulators. Incidentally till 1990 the model F was the most widely used machine in the Indian Armed Forces and were replaced with the Boyle Major. This was manufactured with additional features in mind. These facilities include self-sealing O_2 supply points for operating ventilators, sprays, injector and suction units; combined non-return blow-off valve which opens at 100cmH_2O; swivel outlet which the breathing circuit can be attached and longer flowmeters (230mm long with O_2 range 100ml/min to 8liters/min and N_2O range 200ml/min to 12liters/min). The Boyle MK III and MK IIIS (stainless steel) were available in the market in the 1980's. In these machines the O_2 rotameters are placed downstream and O_2 and N_2O regulators function on the master slave mechanism. The non-return cum pressure relief valve is set 200cm H_2O so that the Manley Servovent Ventilator or IOL Anaesthesia Ventilator MK 1 could be used with the machine. Built in space for a total of 3 vaporizers including Floutec MK 3 is provided. The CO_2 provision has been removed. Boyle MK IV is essentially a MK III machine with provision of essential monitoring equipment namely FiO_2 monitor, end-tidal CO_2, pulse oximeter and ventilation meter. The master slave regulator called nitrolock supplies N_2O only when the minimum supply of O_2 is above 200ml/min. Machine technology has shown tremendous strides in the 90's as pneumatics, electronics and computer science have all been incorporated into the development of the modern anaesthesia machine. Understanding the anatomy of these machines has now become an integral part of the safe practice of Anaesthesia. Boyle 'Tec' and Boyle 'Ultima' are the latest machines being manufactured by IOL in India and are close replicas of the Excel type anaesthesia machines being manufactured in Europe. In the last decade of the last century we have seen a decline in the status of N2O and air as a substitute to N2O has been utilized by many centers. WHO in conjunction with the WFSA have recommended the use of air in lieu of nitrous oxide when volatileanaesthetic agents and balanced anaesthetic technique is employed particularly so for developing countries. The Pedius B anaesthetic machine manufactured by Dragerwerk Germany is one such machine which has an air compressor and oxygen concentrator is quite popular. Usha-Drager a subsidiary of Dragerwerk has started its production in India of a similar apparatus.

IPPV during anaesthesia became a part of the anaesthetic technique with the introduction of muscle relaxants in the armamentarium of anaesthetic drugs. A number of ventilators designed for anaesthetic purposes are available in the Indian market. Few of them are displayed in poster form. Some very handy ventilating devices for use with the Magill's circuit that were used were the minute volume dividers such as Manley, Autovent and Minivent.

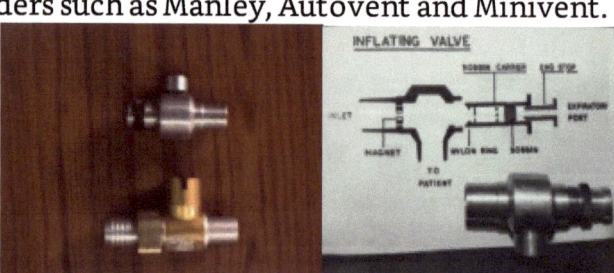

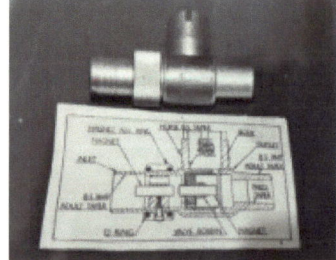

Minivent was considered the smallest ventilators to be ever manufactured and was also known as a discharging compliance ventilator. **Autovent** functions similarly but incorporates two magnets in its functioning as compared to one in the minivent. Line diagrams of both these devices are displayed to help understand their functioning. There was a time when with manual ventilation it was considered better to use non-return valves instead of the Heidbrink type of valves with the Magill's circuit in order to prevent rebreathing.

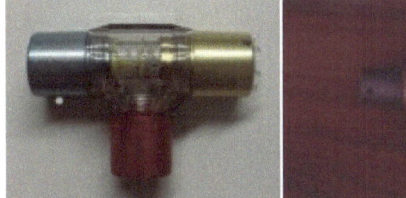

Ruben's valve and **Mitchell's valve** are representatives of such non return valves. The former operates with help of springs and the latter with two magnets.

Vaporizer rather than the word inhaler is used when we are talking of inhalational anaesthesia by continuous flow anaesthetic machines.

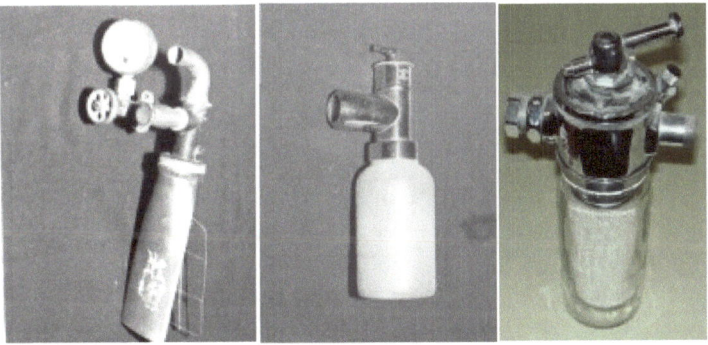

Component parts of some early vaporizers which have not been completely deciphered are also on exhibit. **Bernoy's ether vaporizer, Ogeston's chloroform vaporizer and Ohio N0.8 ether vaporizer** are some of these of vaporizers that could be fitted on different anaesthesia machines in the early 1950's and are available as exhibits.

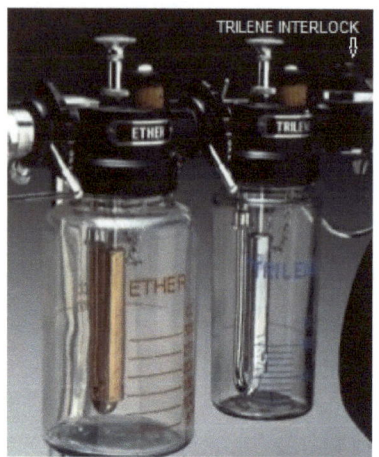

The vaporizers incorporated in the Boyle's Model F were the **Ether and Trilene bottle vaporizers** fitted on the back bar. Both were variable bypass vaporizers. The concentration of ether or trilene could be increased by varying the lever position from off to on. Further increase in concentration could be accomplished by depressing the plunger so that more gas could be bubbled through the liquid and enhance vaporizing interface. A safety feature in the Boyle's machine was the triline interlock. When the unit was put in the closed circuit then trilene vaporizer lever would get locked in the off position or if the lever of the vaporizer was opened then the machine could only be operated in the open circuit position.

A number of stand-alone vaporizers were subsequently developed and could be attached to the outlet of any anaesthesia machine. Some of them are depicted below.

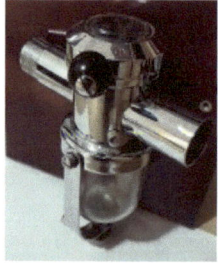

The **Goldman vaporizer** though initially designed for intermittent flow machines dental machines in England. In India and the Armed Forces, it found its maximum utility in continuous flow machines with semi closed circuits. Its use in closed circuit anaesthesia (VIC) in a spontaneously breathing patient has been advocated but we don't see it being used much in this fashion. Its calibration at 30, 8 and 2 lit/min has therefore been done for use in intermittent flow machines, magill's circuit and closed circuit respectively. Till date four versions of the vaporizer have appeared. The Mk IV has four notches and lever for change in concentration has a clicking device.

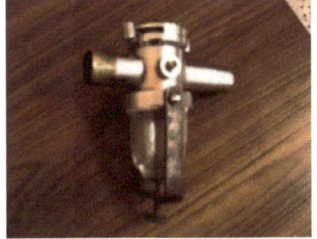

Goldman type vaporizers (eg. Khushwaqt) are prototypes of the same started being manufactured and marketed in India and are akin to the MK IV version.

Some of the next generation vaporizers were the OMV, AE Vaporizer, PDV (penlon draw over vaporizer) and EMO inhaler (already described) . All of these have low internal resistance and can therefore function as draw over vaporizers. Goldman vaporizer too was being used as a draw over vaporizing unit in some portable apparatuses. Another added feature of these vaporizers was that apart from the primary agent these vaporizers incorporated scales for various agents (ether, chloroform, trilene, methoxyflurane, halothane). An ideal vaporizer those days was one that could be used for multiple agents.

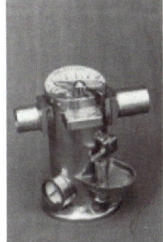

Oxford Miniature Vaporizer (OMV) which was designed for halothane has one scale for trilene. Two versions of OMV exist; OMV

Fifty (Left to Right) for use in continuous flow machines and OMV Ten (Right to Left) for use in draw over anaesthetic apparatus. Facility for temperature stabilisation exist in this vaporiser.

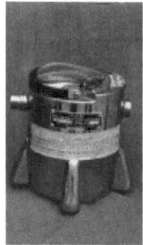

The **AE vaporizer** mfd by 'Cyprane' was designed for halothane but has a dial for chloroform and trilene. It is a temperature compensated vaporizer. Chloroform is probably as good as an anaesthetic as halothane but it fell into disrepute and lost popularity altogether since accurate vaporizers for its delivery did not exist. This vaporizer probably marked the reintroduction of chloroform but never got a foothold.

The **Penlon Draw over Vaporizer (PDV)** which had been designed for methoxyflurane has an additional scale for trilene. It was introduced in Indian Army in the 1960's being considered superior to the EMO. Its use however declined soon after with the withdrawal of methoxyflurane due to its flouride toxicity.

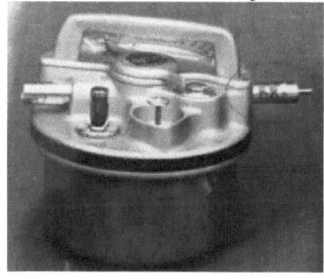

The Epstein, Macintosh, Oxford Inhaler (EMO) apart from ether has a scale for trilene and halothane. It has been mentioned earlier but this picture depicts the famous **'RR' adaptor** attached to its inlet. The adaptor was designed by Brig Rama Rao, Consultant to the Armed Forces way back in 1970. Its use for enrichment of air with oxygen was considered superior to enrichment via the Oxford Inflating Bellows because dilution of ether was prevented. Four versions exist. In Mk IV the chamber was made of stainless steel and control rotor was PTFE coated. Use of a single vaporizer that could be used for other agents was a desirable property of an ideal vaporizer. These days after the introduction of the Tec series we desire to have vaporizers for a single agent.

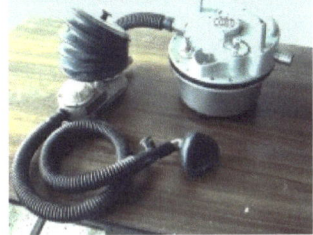

In India portable anaesthetic apparatus e.g. **Oxford inflating bellows in combination with the EMO inhaler** have been popular not only from the private practitioner's point of view but also from the fact that to extend Anaesthesia facilities to the vast rural population this would seem to be the only logical choice. Moreover, the Indian Armed Forces are located in far flung remote areas which may be cut off from the mainstream habitation for days together. Such apparatuses are a great boon in such situations. A notable design of a portable continuous flow anaesthetic apparatus available with the Indian Army is the Field Boyle which is capable of being dropped by parachute in a suitcase like box.

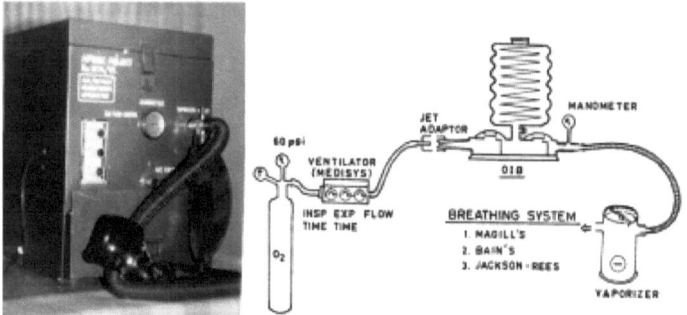

An **air/oxygen continuous flow portable apparatus** using the Oxford Inflating Bellows in conjunction with an indigenous jet ventilator (Medisys) has been designed by the author in 1991 for use in developing countries. Its line diagram, namely the **VOVB** (**V**entilator **O**IB **V**aporizer **B**reathing circuit) is depicted alongside. Basically, it is a reassembly of the existing field equipment in the Indian Armed Forces to achieve a continuous flow of air and oxygen in the event of shortage of nitrous oxide. The system can be used with the various Mapleson circuits.

OXYGEN THERAPY AND RESUSCITATION

The virtues of oxygen though realized by Lavoisier and John Hunter as early as 1774 it was J.S.Haldane who popularized its use during the First World War to resuscitate patients with lung injury as a result of gassing injury. The statement "Oxygen lack not only stops the machine but also wrecks the machinery" is found in almost all text books in medicine and are the words quoted by Haldane. As is evident from the section on anaesthetic apparatus, oxygen was incorporated in the anaesthesia machines only in the second third decade of this century.

Commercial production of oxygen from fractional distillation and storage as liquid oxygen is now being focused to oxygen concentrators (molecular sieves made of artificial zeolite) with a high pressure intensifiers eg. Remer-Alco. Buying in liquid and bottled oxygen can be extremely expensive where transport charges from supplier assume a high proportion of the delivered price. Such devices are also available in portable form eg. Air Sep 4LyF compressed breathing apparatus for ward use. They deliver 95% pure oxygen at flow rates 0-5lit/min and can be stored at <10psi. The only disadvantage being the requirement of constant electric supply. Literature on these devices along with the devices for administering oxygen to spontaneously breathing patients is amply displayed. Though a simple classification of the types of masks used for oxygen therapy could be simple, partial rebreathing, nonrebreathing and those with air entrainment it is better to consider them on a scientific basis as described by Bethune and Collis in 1967. Fixed performance systems are independent of patient factors. In this category fall the high flow air entrainment masks (eg. ventimask) and low flow anaesthetic circuits. The former utilize the venturi principle so that a low flow of oxygen can be used to draw large quantities of air resulting

in a total flow in excess of the peak inspiratory flow. The resulting FiO_2 can be varied from 0.24 to 0.6 in this oxygen enriched air. Variable performance systems (nasal cannula, M.C. mask, polymask, BLB mask, oxygen tent etc.) are largely patient dependent and
can deliver 21-100% O_2 depending upon the interrelationship of oxygen flow, device factors (capacity or no capacity) and patient factors.

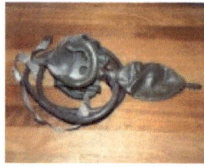

The **BLB** (Boothby, Lovelace, Bulbulian) masks both oral and nasal have somehow still managed to remain in the service hospitals despite the availability of better devices. Nowadays the initial rubber material is now replaced with PVC. Boothby a dental surgeon at the Mayo clinic aero medical unit was a member of the team which included Drs. W. Randolph Lovelace and Walter M. Boothby, which developed the BLB masks which were useful for clinical settings, and, as it turned out, for aviators at high altitudes. They were used in II world war.

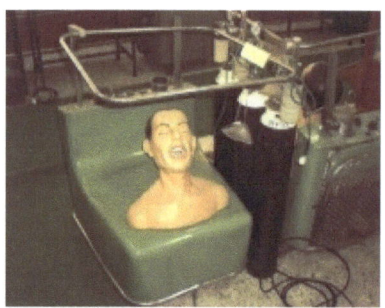
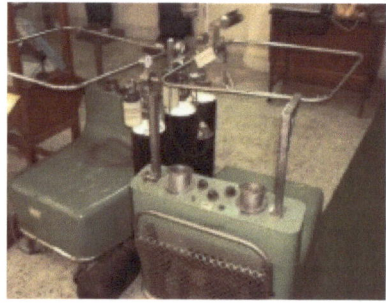

Oxygen tents for adults though popular in the 60's are now only reserved for children as in adults access to the patient gets restricted. Moreover, desired oxygen concentrations are difficult to achieve and the potential fire hazard exists. The oxygen tent exhibited in the museum was manufactured by Oxygenoire Ltd. London.

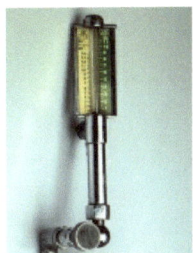

A **Heidbrink flowmeter for He/O$_2$** mixture (80:20) is exhibited. Helium and oxygen have similar viscosities but their densities 0.16 and 1.33 Kg m-3, differ markedly. At low flow rates where the influence of viscosity predominates, helium can be measured with tolerable accuracy on an oxygen rotameter. At high flow rates the effect of density is paramount and the amount of helium delivered by an oxygen rotameter would be almost twice than that indicated. Hence the need for a separately designed flowmeter. He/O$_2$ mixtures are helpful for patients with obstructive lung disease in whom the increased resistance as a result of the narrowing of the air passages causes increased work of breathing. The low density of helium results in less effort to breathe a He/O$_2$ mixture than an air enriched O$_2$ mixture.

Carbon dioxide in the third decade of this century was being extensively used for respiratory emergencies and anaesthetic purposes.

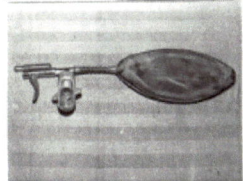

A **sparklet resuscitator** "model C" manufactured by Sparklets Ltd, Upper Edmonton, London during that period is displayed in this section. It comprises of a sparklet holder. a valve key and a rubber reservoir bag and is used for "open" method of CO$_2$ administration. The sparklet bulbs are very similar to the mini bulbs of CO$_2$ used in the modern soda siphons. This device was recommended to be carried in the physician's hand bag.

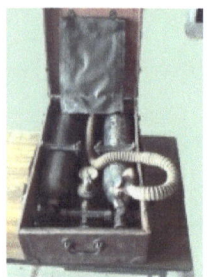

A resuscitation outfit system "**Novalta**" manufactured by Siebe Gormon & Co Ltd, London; probably used during the same period as the sparklet resuscitator utilizes oxygen. It consists of two O_2 cylinders connected to a pressure gauge and dial type flowmeter. Oxygen passes to a rectangular shaped rubber reservoir and then to the patient via a corrugated hose. The face mask is fitted with an air entrainment valve to regulate the percent of O_2 inhaled. The modern inhalational O_2 therapy apparatus eg. Penlon are incorporating demand valves which supply O_2 only during the inspiratory phase and thus prevent wastage. The importance of positive pressure ventilation was recognized only in the 60's.

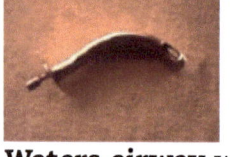

Waters airway was the forerunner of the Guedels airway. It was made of metal and had a side opening in case the distil opening gets obstructed by the soft tongue. The airway has a side port feed for oxygen which is an interesting feature. This was device was in use in the 1920's.

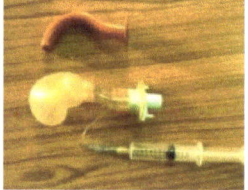

Since then a number of simple devices have found their way for commencing basic life support measures. The Safar Tube, Lifeway, Laerdal pocket mask, Bag-Valve-Mask devices (Vitalograph, Ambu, Laerdal, Sanjeevni and other indigenously manufactured)

and of late a **Cuffed oropharyngeal airway (COPA)** which is in fact a **Guedel Airway** incorporating a cuff can be seen in the exhibits.

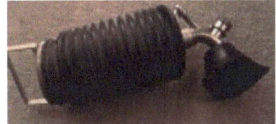

Paediatric resuscitators bellows type (Lala's-Khushwaqt) an alternative to the bag type (Penlon) resuscitators is among the few indigenous devices on display.

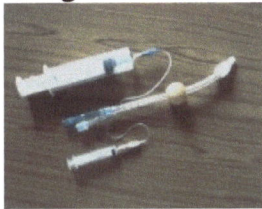

Emergency devices for control of the airway have been devised from time to time for the purposes of resuscitation. The same are also useful when dealing with cases where difficult intubation is anticipated. **Esophageal tracheal combitube (ETC)**, Esophageal obturator airway (EOA), Esophageal gastric tube airway (EGTA), and Laryngeal mask airway (LMA) can be seen as exhibits and posters.

The need for humidification during respiratory therapy was only recognized in 1958 by I.E.Cushings and W.F.Miller in 1958.

The foremost of all humidifier's was the Woulfe bottle (combined bubbling type flowmeter cum humidifier). Though obsolete it continues to be manufactured and used in many places in our country. Basically, a glass bottle with a screw capped metal cover incorporating a hollow tubing which dipped in the water. There were vertically placed single holes on the tube. At the end of the tube were multiple holes. When oxygen was allowed to flow through the bottle then the flow of oxygen could be estimated by seeing through which hole oxygen was bubbling through in the metal tube. If it was from the topmost first hole, the flow was 1Lt/min; if it was from the second hole then flow was 2Lt/min and so on until at multiple holes it was 8Lt/min. A safety valve was incorporated on the metal cap of the bottle which got released when the pressure exceeded 5 lb/sq". Amongst the most sophisticated heated water humidifier's is the one manufactured by Fischer & Paykel. Its advantage is that it produces water vapour without rain out due to its unique servo-controlled heated delivery system.

Development of devices for artificial ventilation have been taking place for the last 150 years or so. Negative pressure ventilators were first introduced by Drinker in 1928. Their pattern of ventilation is like the normal breathing.

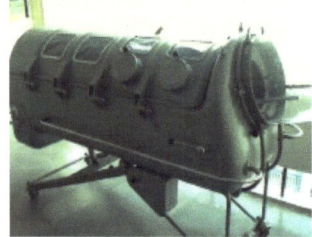

The **Iron lung body tank** is one such ventilator. The "Model E2" manufactured by Dragerwerk, Lubeck; is an all metal impressive looking device which occupies a place at the entrance of the Department. The device completely isolates the patient except the head and working ports are present through which nursing care can be given. The inspiration in this apparatus is caused by an intermittent negative pressure created by an electric motor acting on a piston like device occupying the foot end of the chamber. In cases of power failure, a manual pumping lever helps in creating a negative force for initiating the inspiration.

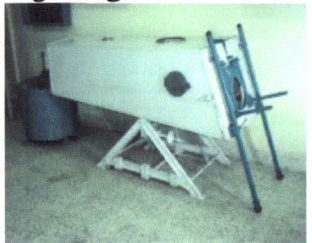

An iron lung made of wood/metal similar to the **Nuffield type cabinet respirator** was developed and manufactured in Armed Forces by the 512 Comd EME W/S Kirkee. No records are traceable to ascertain how efficient this apparatus was nor is there any anaesthesiologist of that period alive to give evidence of its utility.

The body tanks isolated the patients therefore cuirasses or chest shells were designed to allow greater freedom of movement but at the expense of efficiency.

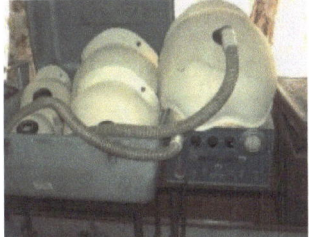

The **Monaghan ventilator** manufactured in Denver, Colorado, U.S.A is one such device. It consists of a rigid shell which is applied to the anterior thoracic and abdominal wall. It contacts the skin at its edges with a padded rubber rim. Five sizes of the shell are provided. A common corrugated hose connects the center of the shell to an electric motor which provides intermittent negative pressure. This device was also recommended about 20 years back for maintaining respiration during general anaesthesia for bronchoscopies. Positive pressure ventilators proved their efficacy over negative pressure ventilators in the Copenhagen polio epidemic of 1952.

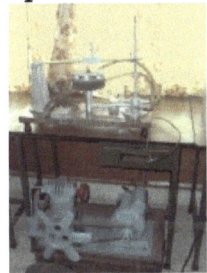

A ventilator similar to the Vellore ventilator which was devised for use as both an anaesthetic and ward ventilator by one of the earlier faculty in the 1970's and came to be known as the AFMC Ventilator. A bulky compressor formed part of the equipment and had very risky fan blades without any protection. Somehow it never went into production due to inherent faults.

A wide variety of conventional positive pressure ventilators were manufactured all over the world in the decades to follow. Pressure cycled ventilators such as the Bennett and Bird series of ventilators were popular in the United States whereas the Engstrom ventilator which was basically volume cycled gained popularity in Europe. In the ARDS era corresponding to the late 1960's most volume cycled ventilators started incorporating PEEP and ability to vary the FiO_2 in their construction (eg. Emerson, Engstrom model 200, Ohio 500, Bennet MAI). With the concept of patient cycling and advent of IMV the 1970's saw the introduction of these techniques in the ventilators of that period.

In the Indian Armed Forces the **East Radcliffe ventilator** a constant pressure device was the popular anaesthesia and ICU ventilator. The ventilator could be used in the circle anaesthesia system or as a non-rebreathing circuit. At the air inlet a draw over vaporizer could be placed so that air-halothane or air-trilene anaesthesia could be administered. PEEP could be added to the IPPV by applying a water seal at the expiratory port of the ventilator. The other ventilator available in the services for use in ICU's was the Bird Mk7. These were phased out in the late 1980's

The new generation of micro-processor controlled mechanical ventilators introduced in the 1980's has eclipsed all manufacturing techniques of the past. The ability to set a ventilator with micro-processor controls has allowed for variation in the pressure wave form with graphic displays. They can be programmed to provide additional assistance, such as SIMV, MMV, I/E Ratio reversal, Pressure support, PEEP, CPAP and APRV. These new modes of ventilation have emerged to tackle the varied and altered pulmonary characteristics of ARDS and also to minimize the work of breathing during weaning from ventilatory support. A wide range of monitoring devices together with several alarm features are part of the machines. Though numerous ventilators are available of the shelf the world over; in India, the CPU-1 of Ohmeda, Bird 2000, Veolar of Hamilton Medical, Drager and the Bear 5 have captured the market.

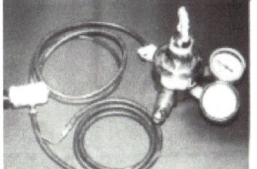

The **venturi Jet (Sanders)** for ventilation was introduced during this period and microlaryngeal surgery in particular was benefited by this technique.

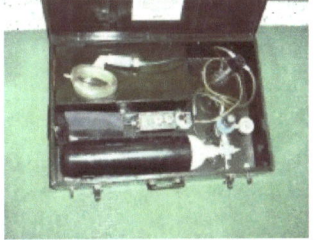

The Bear group introduced a versatile jet ventilator but an indigenous version, the **Medisys System-II** is a very popular ventilator all over the country because of its extremely versatile nature and comparatively low cost. Understandably it uses a source of compressed air or oxygen.

This portable mechanical jet ventilator running under pressurized oxygen is available in the field units of the Armed Forces and is a valuable aid for resuscitation. The unit is indigenously produced by Premier Medical Systems and Devices, New Delhi. The ventilator is provided with a somewhat bulky and noisy compressor when used with compressed air. This being its disadvantageous feature.

Domiciliary ventilators have been marketed and also supplied on rental basis to respiratory cripples for long term ventilation in order to cut down on the finances for the patient and also prevent occupation of an important critical care bed of any institution. Models of Puritan-Bennett, Life Care and Bear products are among the few positive pressure ventilators that have found their way for home care.

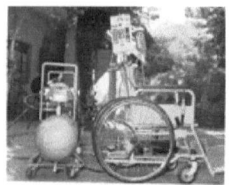

An **indigenous domiciliary wheelchair ventilator** was fabricated by the author for a case of Myasthenia Gravis in 1987. Basically it comprises of the ventilating jet module of the medisys ventilator with an accompanying jet suction fitted onto the vertical bar of the backrest of a wheel chair. Below the wheel chair is fitted an oxygen cylinder which can run the ventilator for six hours at a stretch when the patient is outdoors. Attachment for a compressor are available for use when the patient is indoors. This ventilator was manufactured with the help of Premier Medical Systems and Devices, New Delhi and can form the basis on which home care can be provided under Indian conditions.

Two simple devices for paediatric resuscitation can be described in this section. They are mentioned below.

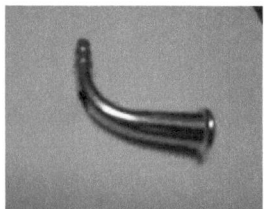

Barrie Connector for resuscitation of Newborn. The smaller diameter end is supposed to be connected to the endotracheal tube and the other end to an oxygen source. The opening on the body of the connector is intermittently closed by a finger to allow intermittent lung inflation.

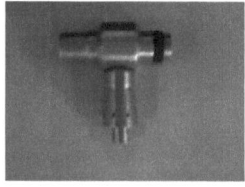

Paediatric leak valve for use with minivent. Modification of adult ventilators for paediatric use can be done by making a parallel compliance system or providing a leak in the inspiratory phase. The leak valve for use in the minivent provides the necessary leak.

ENDOTRACHEAL ANAESTHESIA

All anaesthesiologists are expected to be experts in the art of endotracheal intubation. They are assisted in this complex task by a variety of instruments that allow them to intubate the trachea of patients with even severe anatomical abnormalities that would have been beyond the skill of even the expert practitioners of the past. Endotracheal anaesthesia, as we know it today, is the result of the work of E.S.Rowbotham and Sir Ivan Magill during the years 1917 to 1920. They deserve to be remembered for having simplified and made universally practicable the technique of endotracheal anaesthesia, that they were adopted by anaesthetists throughout the world. Franz Kuhn, a German surgeon during 1900-1912 wrote a number of papers on the art intubation but his works remained untranslated in English and therefore unrecognized by rest of the world for some time. Direct visualization of the larynx by any instrument was probably that devised by Kirstein in 1895 in Berlin and was the forerunner of all the modern laryngoscopes. It was actually a shortened oesophagoscope that was cut anteriorly resulting in a semicircular blade with an anterior concavity. This section deals with not only instruments required for intubation but also the various endotracheal tubes that have evolved over the years together with the ancillary equipment which are necessary for maintaining and supporting a patent airway.

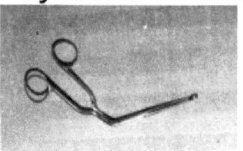

Sir Ivan Magill (1888-1986) the most distinguished pioneers of endotracheal intubation developed techniques of deliberate nasotracheal intubation and as an aid to manipulate the catheter tip, devised the **Magill angulated forceps** in 1920 which still continues to be manufactured without alteration in its design. His technique of positioning the head in the "morning air sniffing position" i.e. the flexion of cervical spine with extension at the atlanto-occipital joint is still in practice.

The **Magills straight blade laryngoscope** designed before the era of muscle relaxants for direct laryngoscopy is no longer favoured when compared with those designed by Robert Miller (U.S.A) and Sir Robert Macintosh (U.K) around 1941. **Miller's blade** is straight with a slightly curved end designed to ease the passage of the tube through the larynx and it is used in a similar fashion as the Magill's blade by lifting the epiglottis in order to expose the larynx.

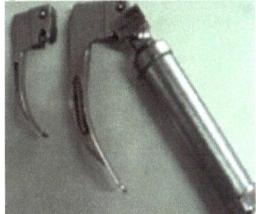

The **Macintosh blade** is curved and its tip is passed in front of the epiglottis and the base of the tongue is lifted resulting in a complete exposure of the laryngeal inlet. The use of this blade prevents stimulation of the vagus and can therefore be used in a lighter plane of anaesthesia without producing laryngeal spasm. Moreover, it gives better exposure and is less traumatic. A wide variety of variations of the Macintosh blade have subsequently been designed to overcome distorted anatomy; some of these are represented in poster form. The Polio blade in which the blade is offset from the handle at an obtuse angle is useful for short necks, obese, mammary hyperplasia, kyphosis, barrel chests and restricted neck movements due to fractures or body jackets. The Huffman Prism laryngoscope is a block of plexiglass shaped to fit onto the proximal end of the Macintosh blade. A refraction of 30 degrees in the line of sight is provided, thereby enabling a better exposure of the larynx in patients in whom it would be difficult otherwise. The image is right side up. The Patil-Syracuse laryngoscope is a Macintosh blade which is adjustable. Four different angles between handle and blade can be achieved. At 45 degrees it is useful for a receding jaw, anterior placed larynx and protruding teeth; at 90 degrees it acts like the conventional laryngoscope; at 135 degrees it serves special nursing needs and at 180 degrees it behaves as the polio blade. The Howland lock is yet another device which fits in between the blade and handles of conventional laryngoscopes and is used to change the angle between the blade and handle.

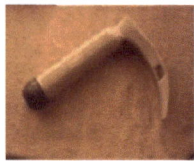

Plastic handle cum blade laryngoscopes (**Penlon**) are now in fashion. The bulbs too are now being incorporated in the handle and the light is being carried forward in the blade by a fibre light bundle. The fibre optic laryngoscope was first described by P. Murphy in 1967. It is an important device for accomplishing intubation under direct vision when it just impossible to even visualize the laryngeal inlet be any means such as bilateral TM joint ankylosis. Components of such a device are a light source; a handle; the body which has the focusing eye piece, working channel sleeve and tip control knob; the flexible insertion portion which consists of a bundle of image-conducting fibres, a bundle of light-conducting fibres and an image forming lens and a tip cable which allows movement of the tip. The device has limitations in that it cannot be used in the paediatric age group because of the fixed diameter of the flexible insertion portion. A wide range of straight blades for neonates and infants have been recommended as they can lift the longer epiglottis, though many would continue to prefer the smallest sized Macintosh blade.

The Seward, Robertshaw, Oxford, Wisconsin, Anderson, Scadwell and Oxyscope are some common names which one comes across. It is generally the flange of the blade which is modified in some way or the other.

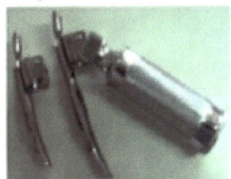

The **Oxyscope** is essentially a Miller's blade that has an attachment that allows delivery of oxygen thus preventing desaturation during intubation. This is particularly useful for neonates during awake intubation. The Anderson laryngoscope has a hook on the handle which can be used to hold the handle with the help of the index finger. Though metal endotracheal tubes were designed as early as 1885 by Joseph O'Dwyer to treat patients in diphtheritic crisis their use in anaesthesia was largely due to the efforts of Sir Ivan Magill who in a hardware store found several sizes of mineralized red rubber tubing which he cut, beveled and smoothed to produce tubes that clinicians in all countries would come to call "Magills tubes". Till the 1960's endotracheal tubes continued to be made of rubber when inert plastics started taking its place. The cuff in endotracheal tubes was as a result of the genius of Arthur Guedel (1883 to 1956). He fashioned cuffs from the rubber of dental dams, condoms and surgical gloves that were glued onto the outer wall of tubes. After a series of animal experiments, he recommended that the position of the cuff be positioned below the level of the vocal cords. Ralph Waters later recommended that cuffs be constructed of two layers of soft rubber cemented along the edge. Some tubes being manufactured incorporate two cuffs. In one the cuffs are located one above the other and in another one inside the other. The advantage is that in case of damage to one the other may by used. The former type is also recommended during prolonged intubation when the cuffs are inflated in an alternate fashion so that mucosal trauma is minimized. There has been a tendency after 1970 to have high-volume low-pressure cuffs as they offer greater protection against cuff induced complications after prolonged intubation. For short term intubations the older high pressure low-volume cuffs do offer certain advantages (better visibility during intubation, better protection against aspiration, lower incidence of sore throats and be able to be used repeatedly). There is widespread belief that simply using high volume low-pressure cuffs will prevent high pressures being exerted on the wall of the trachea. This is only true if such cuffs are not over inflated when dangerously high pressures can develop; the recommended intra-cuff pressure being approximately 20-30 torr. At this pressure aspiration is prevented and at the same time mucosal perfusion ensured.

Turbomat is one such device that helps to monitor and maintain intra-cuff pressure and ought to be used whenever high-volume low-pressure cuffs are used. The pressure is adjusted when airway pressure is least (i.e. at end expiration during IPPV or peak inspiration during spontaneous respiration). Foam/Sponge cuffs (Kamen-Wilkinson) described in 1970 have a large diameter and residual volume. These types of cuffs comprise of polyurethane foam covered with a sheath. Applying suction to the inflating tube causes the foam to contract. When the negative pressure is released after tube insertion the cuff expands and the pressure in the cuff remains atmospheric.

These cuffs have all the virtues high pressure or low pressure cuffs but the optimal size tubes are required to achieve the purpose. Detachable cuffs are now available for use with silver tracheal tubes which are being recommended for laser surgery. Some tubes have a hole near the patient end one on the side opposite the bevel. This is known as Murphy's eye and its purpose is to allow gases to pass if the bevel is occluded. Such Murphy tubes date back to the year 1941. Most of the modern tubes incorporate this eye during manufacture. The design of bevel for oral or nasal use has now been superseded by tubes called oro-nasal tubes that can be used for either oral or nasal use. The presence of a cuff in an endotracheal tube has the additional advantage of keeping the tube centrally in the trachea thereby preventing the bevel from irritating the tracheal wall. During neurosurgery in patients posi-

tioned with the head in acute flexion it is possible for the bevel to abut against the tracheal wall to cause occlusion. There has been a tendency to cut the terminal end of Oxford tubes to eliminate the bevel altogether especially in the uncuffed Oxford tubes. The description of the cuffs, bevels described above have been amply illustrated in the plates displayed in this section. Ever since the introduction of the red rubber tubes known
popularly as the Magill's tubes a wide range of endotracheal tubes in material and design have been manufactured to achieve characteristics such as lack of toxicity, transparency, smooth and non wettable, non kinkable, thermoplastic and non-reactive with lubricants and anaesthetic agents. To suit individual needs. The plethora of tubes now available and their flooding the market has created complexities for a buyer. Broadly the materials utilized for manufacture are Rubber (red or white); Plastics (PVC, PVC clear, PVC Ivory, PVC siliconized); Latex with or without silicon and Silicon rubber. The main concern in the material used for manufacture is the evidence of tissue toxicity. The markings "IT" or "Z-79" on a tube is evidence that the tube material has been tested and and no evidence of toxicity has been found. Prominent manufacturers of endotracheal tubes abroad are Portex Ltd, Willy Rusch, National Inc, Mallinckrodt Inc. and Euromedical. All these companies have their representatives in India. Romsons is the only Indian based firm manufacturing inexpensive endotracheal tubes of reasonably fair quality. However, "The best buy for endotracheal tubes" is illustrated in a chart and is very comprehensive.

Special tubes to suit individual needs and for different anaesthetic techniques have been designed from time to time. Some of them are mentioned and the requisite literature or samples are displayed. For convenience sake they have been grouped under various categories.

CATEGORY OF TUBES

1.Preformed tracheal tubes: RAE (Ring-Adiar- Elwyn) or Polar tubes which are available as South or North (oral/nasal), Oxford tubes, Teheran tube.

2.Special function tubes: Endotrol / Tracheal tube with controllable tip, Gas monitoring tube (Deane), Laser-Shield tracheal tube that is impregnated with metal particles, Micro laryngeal surgery tubes (Simple cuffed 4-5mm internal diameter tubes up to 40cm long, Hi-Lo Jet tracheal tubes having 3 lumens, Injectoflex), Motando tube, plain silver tubes with detachable cuffs. Oxford right angle tubes with or without bevel /cuff for paediatric/adult use.

3.Double lumen tubes: Carlen's red rubber or PVC, White, Robertshaw, Bryce-Smith.

4.Paediatric tubes:

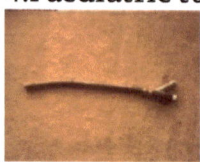

The **Magills Flexometallic** described by Magill was as early as 1934. It was a modified T piece soldered onto a spring over which was slipped on a rubber sheath.

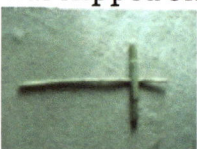

JacksonRees T-tube which incorporates its own T-piece and suction facility.

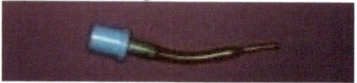

Cole tube was designed for neonatal resuscitation. The 3.0 mm tube has shoulders at it proximal where the tube becomes a 4.5mm ID tube. This is intended to abut against the laryngeal inlet and prevent the tube from being introduced too deeply, ensuring inadvertent endobronchial intubation.

A fogarty venous embolectomy catheter is also displayed with the paediatric tubes because of its usefulness as a bronchial blocker for OLV in the paediatric age group.

5.Armoured/Reinforced tubes: Metal wire (Flexometallic) or Nylon filaments are embedded in the manufacturing material generally latex or PVC. Nylon reinforced tubes may be preformed with a curvature.

6. Special Devices useful after failed intubation or managing a difficult airway: EOA, EGTA, ETC, COPA have been mentioned in the section on resuscitation but their diagrammatic representation is depicted in this section. The Laryngeal Mask manufactured by Intavent International S.A. is available in four sizes and its preparation, insertion, maintenance and removal are described in the chart displayed.

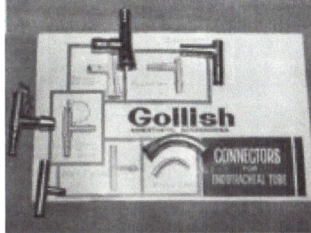 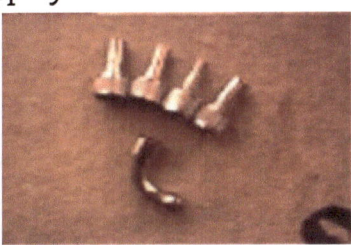

A large number of **Endotracheal tube connectors** which help to connect the endotracheal tubes to the breathing system via a catheter mount were designed by various workers, ever since Magill designed the metal oral and nasal connectors. Samples of the **Magill** (oral and nasal), **Rowbotham**, **Magill suction union**, **Cobb's suction union**, T piece and **Noseworthy** connections are displayed as above.

Various designs of **endotracheal tube connections for paediatric use** were manufactured from time to time; largely with the aim of reducing the apparatus dead space and to have a universal adapter to fit various size tubes.

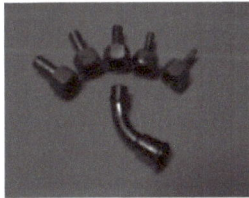

Noseworthy (Knight)

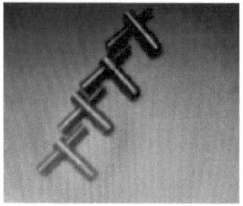

Rendell Baker, made of aluminium to make the connection lightweight.

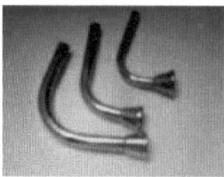

Worcestor type, designed to be extralong so that the endotracheal tube is not compressed when the Doughty mouth gag is applied during tonsillectomy

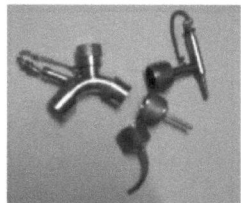

Khushwaqt Pattern, to fit with Chandigarh comprehensive paediatric set (Magill, Noseworthy, Cobb's)

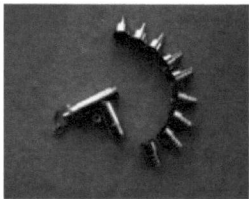

Varanasi set, basically a Cobb's suction union with multiple size attachments for various size endotracheal tubes from paediatric to adult (to fit 3mm to 9mm tubes) was designed in India. Most of these connections were manufactured in India by Khushwaqt industries under ISI specification. Now, however the trend is to use plastic disposable connectors which are generally supplied along with the endotracheal tubes.

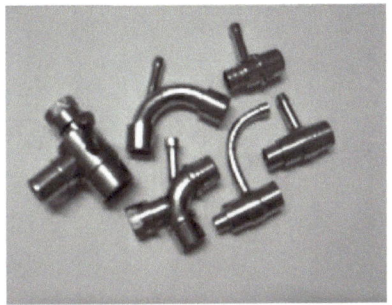

Modified T pieces were designed by various workers to help in convenience of attaching paediatric circuits. The designs have varied for several reasons. 1) Making the main body curved to diminish resistance of airflows. 2) Incorporation of low resistance expiratory valve for making the paediatric circuit more versatile by converting it into a Mapleson A circuit 3) Direction of fresh gas flow to increase or decrease expiratory resistance 4) patient end adopted to directly fit on an endotracheal connector. The Curved mount with side feed, Rendell Baker T piece, MIE / Chandigarh Comprehensive T pieces and T pieces with gas flow inlet in vertical, slanting directions and the extra-long curved gas flow inlet of Wright are displayed.

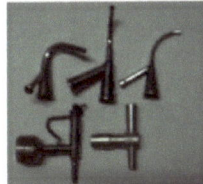

'**T Connectors**' were connections to make the system lighter and incorporate the virtues of the T pieces and endotracheal connectors many paediatric anaesthesiologists had designed connectors as shown above.

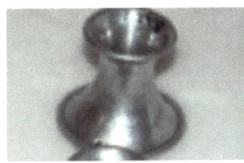 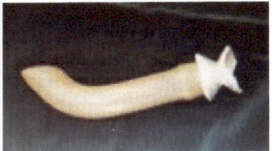

Other ancillary devices such as the **dental props** (**London Hospital pattern**, Adams), Airways (Guedel, Waters, **Hewitts**, Phillips), various types of laryngeal sprays (Macintosh, Rowbotham, Swerdlow) are grouped together in this section.

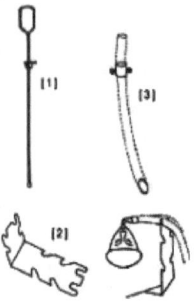

The **adjustable stylet** (1) could be used for a range of endotracheal tubes, **tube tree** (2) was helpful in supporting various types of breathing circuits in different age groups and **endotracheal tube harness's** (3) **for** fixing different size endotracheal tubes. The last was particularly useful in bearded persons. All these accessories had been designed by the author in an attempt to make intubation a safer technique. They are also displayed in this section.

REGIONAL ANAESTHESIA

The credit of introduction of local analgesia goes to Carl Koller (1857-1944) with his experiments with cocaine for ophthalmic surgery in 1884 in Vienna. In the same year the efficacy of the drug was shown over the mucosa of the upper airways, urethra, and rectum in America and by December the same year it was utilized by William Halstead and Richard Hall for blocking of nerves. Soon in 1885, Leonard Corning, a neurologist produced a neurological blockade in a dog by injecting it in the spinal canal. It was he who coined the word "Spinal Anaesthesia". The correct technique of lumbar puncture was described by Hienrich Quincke of Kiel. August Bier a colleague of Quincke performed the first deliberate cocainization of the spinal cord in man in 1899. Surprisingly Bier lost interest in spinal anaesthesia due to the high incidence of complications following lumbar puncture (probably because of use of wide bore needles and non-observance of aseptic techniques) and toxic reactions attributed to cocaine. Though Captain Fidel Pages of the Spanish Army described peridural anaesthesia in 1921 it was Dogliotti of Turin, Italy who wrote a classic in 1931 on the epidural technique utilizing the loss of resistance technique. There have been a large number of workers who have described specific techniques/devices or otherwise contributed to the spread of analgesic solutions in the cerebro-spinal canal. Subarachnoid block has been taught widely only after since 1950's and a systematic study on extradural anaesthesia began only in the 1960's as a result of the work of Bromage. Use of narcotics to produce selective analgesia by these routes was described by Cousins in 1979. Newer and safer local anaesthetic agents are now available (see next section). As far as the needles for spinal and epidural work is concerned the focus has been on the size (SWG), tip shape and position of the needle opening. There has also been a tendency to mark the needles and incorporation of plastic material in the components of needles designed for once use only. In general, the spinal needles are 3 1/2" in length and vary from 25 to 22 gauge though finer needles (up to 32 S.W.G.) to completely abolish chances of CSF leakage and post spinal headache are being manufactured. The use of fine needles, entails the need for some form of introducer as the needle is easily distorted and bent due to increased pliability. For 22 gauge needles we commonly use the blood transfusion needle as the introducer. The only problem with such needles is that it takes longer time for CSF fluid to track back through the needle. Short bevels for spinal needles are desirable as with longer bevels there are chances of incomplete dural punctures. Two, different tip configurations of spinal needle exist. The lancet tip or the cutting bevel (Pitkin) and the pencil point or the non-cutting bevel (Green/Whittaker). The latter parts rather than cuts the duramater. Quincke designed a spinal needle of the lancet type bevel which spreads rather than cuts the longitudinal fibers of the dura. B. Braun is manufacturing such type of needles. Of late 28 gauge styletted microcatheters for rapid and controlled continuous spinal anaesthesia are available (Portex). Epidural needles are of 16 or 18 S.W.G., as with finer needles the loss of resistance technique is not well appreciated. Moreover, these sizes allow the passage of catheters. Two needles are popular ; the Crawford and Tuohy. In the former the risk of dural puncture is reduced and, in the latter, the epidural space is better appreciated. Both spinal and epidural needles may have attached wings (Macintosh) or large spool type hubs to ostensibly facilitate handling of the needle. Most needles come with the calibration advocated by Lee.

Combined spinal/epidural set manufactured by Portex provides rapid onset spinal anaesthesia with the subsequent flexibility of epidural anaesthesia via a catheter. Some of the newer portex products are displayed in poster form.

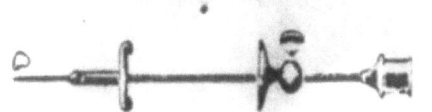

The **spinal needle of Corning** which appeared in Medical Record, 1900, Oct.20.601, is depicted in the above photo. The needle made of gold/platinum had an introducer a sliding nut with a screw to act as a distance marker. Later needles were thick and clumsy and never matched the well thought of and designed needle of Leornard Corning. The very considerable advances in the armamentarium of general anaesthesia has reduced the necessity for the application of conduction analgesia techniques. It is however unjustifiable to even consider that these techniques are no longer valid as there are definite indications in emergency surgery, day case surgery, certain special surgical operations and in patients with intercurrent diseases (cardiac, respiratory, diabetes, uraemia etc.). With this in mind posters were prepared for certain regional techniques which would be useful to any practicing anaesthetist of today. Certain blocks such as inguinal, intercostal, cervical, brachial, laryngeal, subarachnoid and epidural are well illustrated.

DRUGS CONCERNING ANAESTHESIOLOGISTS

With the increased complexity and sophistication of modern drug therapy, it is becoming virtually impossible for any individual to acquire complete knowledge of the actions and potential hazards of all available therapeutic agents. This poses a particularly difficult problem for the anaesthetist, since the drugs employed in anaesthetic practice cover an unusually wide spectrum of compounds of diverse structure, physical and pharmacological properties.

I remember taking few chapters in pharmacology less seriously during my second MBBS. All these chapters surprisingly were very essential from the anaesthetists' point of view and had someone told me during those days about the exciting history and fascinating actions of the gases; narcotics, sedatives and tranquilizers; volatile anaesthetics; local anaesthetics and muscle relaxants I would have been a keen observer of how anaesthesia was administered during the clinical tenure of my training as a doctor. One chapter which I feel that was largely neglected was that connected with fluids/electrolytes and blood transfusion therapy. The real usefulness of blood/plasma components and plasma substitutes was realized after becoming an anaesthetist. My personal feeling is that to be a good anaesthetist one has to have a good working knowledge of 3P's (Physiology, Physics, Pharmacology).

What concerns the anaesthetist more is not the action of a particular drug but how their actions differ in various age groups, in various disease states and in people with different medication. Drug interactions amongst various drugs therefore forms an important consideration when planning the administration of any anaesthetic. The anaesthetists role as a physician to the surgeon requires not only the knowledge of anaesthetic drugs but a wider account of drugs used in general medicine. With the increasing role of anaesthetists as intensivists or critical care specialists the scope has been widened further. Total parenteral nutrition is one of the very essential part of training for a critical care specialist. Today, not only are there drugs which have been reformulated to achieve a specific action but the drug delivery systems have also been refined and made sophisticated. The object of making a section on anaesthetic drugs and drugs concerning anaesthetist is therefore obvious. The grouping and orientation of drugs is purely from the practical and examination point of view. Many drugs may be obsolete but never the less are required to be known to a post graduate student. The drugs of recent origin are not been mentioned basically because they are not easily available in the country and our experience in their usage is lacking. This should not deter any student from not acquiring any knowledge of a particular drug. Samples of the following drugs are displayed. Again, the method of classification is purely from the examination or utility point of view.

List of Drugs on Display

1. Intravenous anaesthetic agents.
(Thiopentone, Methohexitone, Amylobarbitone, Phenobarbitone, Propanadid, Althesin,
Droperidol, Haloperidol, Etomidate, Ketamine, Diazepam, Lorazepam, Propofol)
2. Inhalational anaesthetic agents.
(Nitrous Oxide, Chloroform, Ether, Ethyl chloride, Trilene, Penthrane, Halothane, Isoflurane, Sevoflurane, enflurane, desflurane)
3. Muscle relaxants.
(Tubocurare, Gallamine, Pancuronium, Vecuronium, Atracurium, Rocuronium, Suxamethonium, Methocarbamol)
4. Narcotic Analgesic agents and their antagonists.
(Morphine, Pethidine, Pentazocine, Buprenorphine, Fentanyl, Lethidrone, Noloxone)
5. Drugs acting on the Autonomic nervous system.
(Atropine, Hyoscine, Glycopyrrolate, Neostigmine, physostig-

mine, 4-aminopyridine)
6. Local anaesthetics.
(Lignocaine, Bupivacaine, Dibucaine, Chlorprocaine, Procaine, Etidocaine, EMLAcream)
7. Vasopressors.
(Adrenaline, Nor-adrenaline, Dopamine, Dobutamine. Mephentine, Ephedrine, Methoxamine, Amphetamine, Phenylephrine)
8. Anti-hypertensives.
(Sod Nitroprusside, Nitroglycerine, Trimetaphan, Captopril, Nifedipine, Dilziam, Phentolamine,
Pentolinium, Mag sulphate, Clonidine)
9. Inotropic drugs.
(Digitalis, Dobutamine, Isoprenaline)
10.Other cardiovascular drugs.
(Propranalol, Esmolol, Veramapil, Aldomet, Procainamide, Lignocaine, Phenytoin, Bretylium,
Calcium gluconate/chloride, Potassium chloride)
11.Diuretics
(Frusemide, Mannitol)
12.Anti-asthma drugs.
(Aminophylline, Deriphylline, Etofyline, Hydrocortisone, Dexamethasone, aerosols : steroid/micronephrin/salbutamol/ipratropium)
13.Obstetric drugs.
(Methylergometrine, Oxytocin, Isoxpurine, Prostaglandin-E2)
15.Fluids/Electrolytes/Plasma expanders/ fluids for TPN
(5%Dextrose, 0.9%Isotonic Saline, Hypertonic saline, IGS/dextrose-saline, Ringer Lactate, Hypertonic saline, 7.5/8.4% Sodabicarbonate, Pot chloride, 25%/50% Dextrose, Haemaccel, Dextran in saline/dextrose, Dried pooled Plasma, Fresh Frozen Plasma, aminosol, intralipids,
multivitamins)
14.Miscellaneous drugs.
(Heparin, Protamine, Insulin, Cimetidine, Ranatidine, Metoclopramide, Omeprazole,
Trimeprazine, Promethazine, Chlorpramazine, p-aminomethyl

Benzoic acid, Doxapram, Analgin, Ketorolac, Ascorbic acid, Vitamin K, Hyaluronidase, Phenoxybenzamine, Papaveratum)

A large number of drugs which are of no doubt useful to anaesthesiologists may not have been listed. This is so because of the unavailability of the drug in India (e.g. dantrolene, remifentanyl) or because it has not found its way in the Indian Pharmacopia.

ANAESTHETIC ANCILLARIES

Though a vast number plastic cannula for intravenous use are now available in the market the important factor in their use is how inert the manufacturing material is and how long it can comfortably be kept in the patient. No doubt they have superseded the metal needles as the venous patency is assured and can be kept in situ for a longer duration causing less discomfort to the patient. Scalp vein (butterfly) needles though initially designed for paediatric use are now available in larger sizes and are equally popular because of their lower cost. Life saving central venous catheters of different types (see section on monitoring) are indicated in a surgery where excessive blood loss is anticipated or in situations when no peripheral veins are accessible. Two items of historical interest in this section are the Gordh's needle and the Martin's Pump (manufactured by Khushwaqt). The former was popular when intermittent intravenous anaesthesia was contemplated, so that clotting in the intravenous needle is prevented. Its use was no longer felt with the availability of intravenous infusion sets. The latter was a convenient way for rapid infusion of plasma/blood by a manual method.

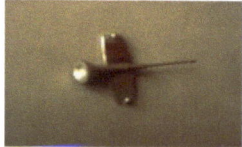

The **Gordh's Needle** was popular in the 1950's. It had a rubber diaphragm through which injections could be given intermittently. These needles were repeatedly used after autoclaving. Needles were sharpened by rubbing on stone.

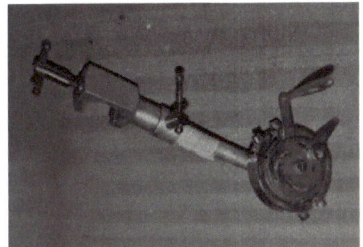

Martin's Pump is a manual pump which employs the roller pump mechanism and has a handle to rotate the rollers. It was useful for rapid transfusion. It was ideal to use sets with rubber tubing, that was placed between the rollers and margin of the bracket. Now electric versions of similar pumps are available and allow the use of PVC tubing.

The "**RR Tray Preset**" designed by Brig Rama Rao, Consultant anaesthetist to the Armed Forces and manufactured by Khushwaqt Industries around 1970 is a compact tray and of good utility for practicing anaesthesiologists. It is a very convenient tray which can accommodate the commonly used drug ampoules, bowl for distilled water/saline and loaded drug syringes. The tray can be autoclaved after use. Fluid and blood giving intravenous sets are now being extensively manufactured in our country. Microdrip (60 drops/ml) sets for giving drugs by infusion and for paediatric use should be selected on the appropriate occasion. Where financial resources are enough one should not hesitate to procure the accurate infusion pumps. These pumps are now being used more and more intraoperatively by anaesthesiologists for giving intravenous anaesthetics, narcotics and relaxants in infusion form.

In the early 1970's an **indigenous infusion pump** designed by Brig Palnitkar (one of the earlier faculty) was one of the earliest pumps designed in India. Apparatuses for intraoperative blood salvage and transfusion are being made available in many theatre complexes in Western countries for intraoperative autotransfusion.

MONITORING & MONITORING EQUIPMENT

Who is the ideal Anaesthetist?

To me a Safe anaesthetist should be considered ideal. A similar view would probably be held by any patient who has not experienced anaesthesia earlier. But, a patient who has undergone the agony/pleasant experience of anaesthesia like my wife, says that an ideal anaesthetist should be one who allows one to wake up with the freshness of the morning air.

During the days when I was doing my post-graduation when there were no real time monitors, alarms my teacher taught me to be alert with five modalities during anaesthesia to be a safe anaesthesiologist 1) Oxygen flow in the flowmeters 2) Movement of the rebreathing bag 3) Finger on the Pulse 4) Color (nail beds/lips) 5) Flow in the Intravenous set. These were probably considered the bare minimum a person could do.

Risks associated with anaesthetic practice have been acknowledged since the introduction of anaesthetic agents as the production of unconsciousness in itself, has, and always will have an element of danger to it. Although some anaesthesiologists began to measure and record pulse and blood pressure during surgical procedures at the turn of the century, in most hospitals intraoperative monitoring for the first hundred years of anaesthesia involved little more than the depth of anaesthesia by observing patterns of respiration, muscle tone, pupillary changes, movement and skin colour.

A sketch of **"The Ideal Anaesthetist"** displayed in this section was distributed by Albury Instruments (see below) and is probably the version of an ideal anaesthetist given by a teacher of anaesthesia. I had seen this sketch during my days as resident in anaesthesia. With so many hands to work with and so much involvement of the special sense organs for the safe conduct of anaesthesia involves tremendous load on the brain. I get quite amused to see the extra hand displayed for pinching the nurses' bottom and presume that this is the essence of humour necessary for making a versatile anaesthetist. A closer look at the sketch will reveal that the anaesthesiologist of today doesn't require so many hands because of the availability of versatile anaesthesia workstations and multiparameter monitors. In fact, an additional Wi-Fi antenna is now available all the time.

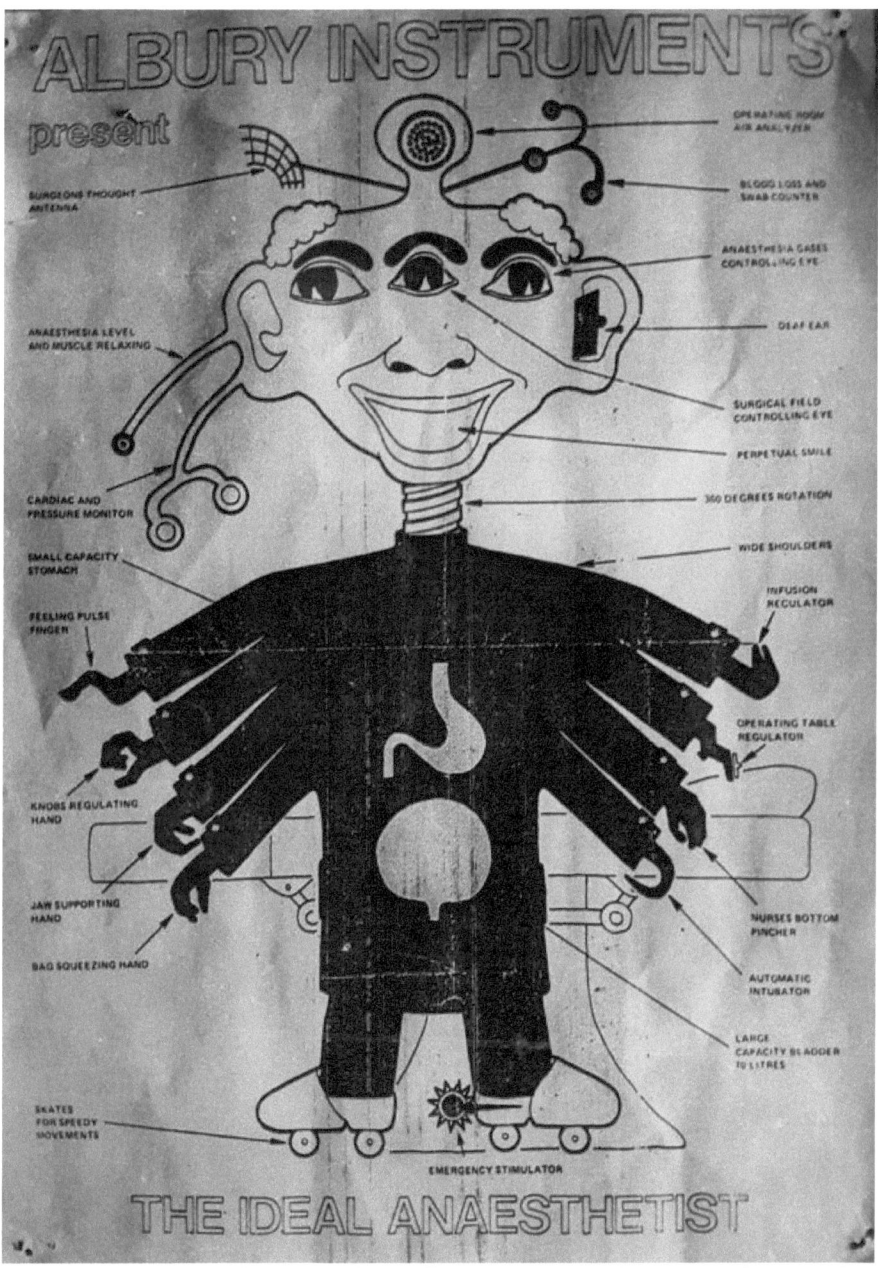

A number of studies to identify and quantify the risks involved in anaesthetizing patients and to recommend definite strategies had lacked uniformity till two to three decades ago. Monitoring cardiovascular, respiratory and muscle relaxation properties were being attempted earlier and many ingenious equipment in the department bear witness to this fact. Risks associated with anaesthetic practice have been acknowledged since the introduction of anaesthetic agents as the production of unconsciousness in itself, has, and always will have an element of danger to it. Monitoring cardiovascular, respiratory and muscle relaxation properties was being attempted earlier and many ingenious equipment now kept as antiques in the department bear witness to this fact. Electronic stethoscopes, pulse meters, ECG machines, Wright's respirometer, oesophageal stethoscope, are among the more antique devices exhibited.

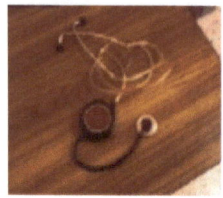 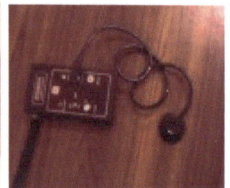

Electronic stethoscopes had become popular in the 1980's. They were particularly useful in amplifying the heart sounds during paediatric anaesthesia.

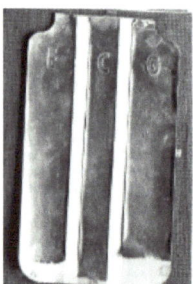

A **Cardiomat ECG electrode** which is 12"x6" cardboard with three silver strips on it is a useful device for use in ECG monitoring where the object is to observe the rate, rhythm, consistency and changes in patient heart action. It does not require fixing the electrodes on to the patient but simply sliding it under the back of the patient.

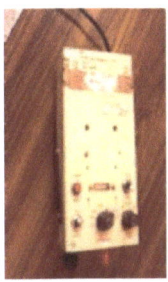

Neuromuscular monitoring was also being attempted based on basic physiology of the nerve muscle preparation we saw in our physiology practical's. The **relaxometer** was a devise in attempting to assess the degree of relaxation based on chronaxie and rheobase. It was the ingenuity of Col RM Mathur one of the earlier faculty to develop such a gadget. Subsequently simple peripheral nerve stimulators were developed before the advent of accelographs and TOF Gaurd. Nowadays we have better devices for monitoring the twitch, TOF and DB.

Out dated very bulky monitors but nevertheless considered to be the discovery of that era were procured for research purposes in the department. Some of them are housed here.

They are the gas chromatograph, blood volume computer (Volemetron) and Osmometer which date back to the sixth decade of the last century.

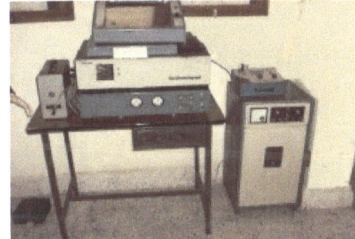

This **Gas chromatograph** was manufactured by Toshniwal Ltd. in 1973 on commercial scale with design developed by Bhaba Atomic Research Centre, Bombay. A bulky equipment consisted of an analyzer oven which has the flame ionization detector, thermal conductivity detector and electron capture detector; temperature controller; electrometer and potentiometric recorder. Its main use was to detect trace anaesthetics and calibration of vaporizers.

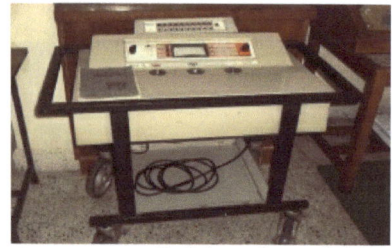

Automated blood volume computer (**Volemetron**) manufactured by Ames Co. Indiana. in 1968. This apparatus was used to determine blood volume perioperatively by adding radioactive tracers (radio-iodinated human serum albumin or Cr51 tagged red cells) to the blood stream and determining the dilution of these tracers in the blood. The results took about 20 minutes to be determined Somehow such devices never became popular.

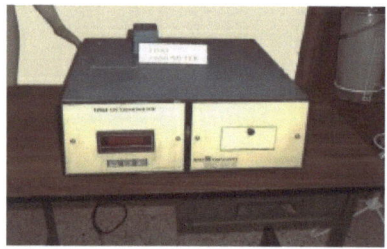

The **Osmometer** manufactured by Fiske Associates, Massachusetts. Procured by the department in 1977 this apparatus helped to determine the osmolarity of blood and urine by measuring their depression of freezing point. The equipment directly displays the units in milliosmoles/Kg.

Though an International Symposium on Preventable Anaesthetic Morbidity and Mortality in 1984 did not achieve any uniformity in monitoring amongst anaesthesiologists, it did pave the way for a thinking on the correct lines. The Department of Anaesthesiology at Harvard published its own monitoring standards in 1986, and similar minimal monitoring standards were adopted by the American Society of Anaesthesiologists (ASA) on October 21 1986. The primary emphasis of these standards for basic monitoring are to ensure that (1) qualified personnel be physically present throughout the anaesthetic care and (2) oxygenation, ventilation, circulation, and temperature be continually (repeated regularly and frequently) or continuously (without interruption) evaluated. The guidelines do not mention specific assessments of renal function, cardiovascular pump function, oxygen utilization, neuromuscular blockade, CNS function, anaesthetic gas concentration or appropriate laboratory support, despite their apparent usefulness.

A review of equipment suitable for minimal monitoring are displayed in poster form. The FiO2 analyser (eg. Ohio 5100), pulse oximeter (e.g. Ohmeda Biox III), capnography (e.g. Ohmeda 5200), electrocardiography (eg.BPL-India), continually monitoring device for blood pressure (eg. dinamap), continuous pulse monitor (Murray-mie) and continuous auscultation of heart/breath sounds (eg. oesophageal stethoscope), continuous temperature monitor with separate probes (skin, oesophagus, rectal) are equipment which one could consider as part minimal monitors required for any anaesthetic procedure.

Noninvasive monitoring has improved dramatically in the past decade and the practice of anaesthesia will become increasingly safer as complications due to invasive techniques will decline. Noninvasive continuous blood pressure monitors and cardiac monitors for automated ST-segment analysis, cardiac output estimation and left ventricular function are now in the market. Two-dimensional Transoesophageal Echocardiography (TEE) is the most complex, expensive but potentially revealing cardiovascular monitor to be introduced.

Posters of neuromuscular blockade monitors (e.g. accelograph, myograph 2000), respiratory data display unit (eg. Mediman), anaesthetic concentration monitors (eg. Gas chromatograph HP8590A, gas monitor type-1304 Bruel and Kjaer, spectrometer Advantage 2000, lamtec 990IMS-Integrated monitoring systems), continuous intravascular oxygen monitoring (e.g. Continucath 1000TM-Biomedical Sensors) and transcutaneous O_2 & CO_2 monitors (eg. Allied Instrumentation Laboratory, Novametrix), ventricular function monitors for cardiac performance (e.g. L&T Medical, 2d-ECHO and Doppler ultrasound), central venous pressure (eg. cavafix) and pulmonary artery pressure (e.g. Swan

Ganz-Gould) monitoring ancillaries and lastly cerebral electrical activity monitoring namely EEG, evoked potentials (eg. Dr.Richard Wiess neuromonitor, ABM-Datex) are few monitoring devices though not listed as essential monitors are useful in their own right depending on the nature of surgery contemplated.

Invasive monitoring was being considered for anaesthesia whenever patients were at poor risk, had associated cardiac problems or when hypotensive techniques were envisaged. Central venous catheters including Swan Ganz catheters can be seen in this section. Old variety of pressure transducers for intra-arterial monitoring and catheters for intra-aortic balloon pumping are on display. With electronic and computer industry shaking hands with the anaesthesiologist a greater degree of automation is coming up and anaesthesia can be administered with greater accuracy and with more proficiency. Software's for drug InfoBase and drug interaction in anaesthesia /critical care; pharmacokinetic and pharmacodynamic drug profiles of intravenous anaesthetics & muscle relaxants along with essential intraoperative data monitoring have paved the way for the development of automated anaesthesia techniques. In the new millennium we are now venturing to monitor other parameters rather than those laid down by Harvard Medical School. However, it must not be forgotten that we belong to the group of developing countries where the financial crunch will force us to continue relying upon our fingers and special senses for the safe conduct of anaesthesia.

Though sterilization of instruments, linen and other articles is not done by anaesthesiologists and is looked after by a CSSD (Central Sterile Supply Department in any hospital; in the Armed Forces the CSSD and its efficiency is monitored by the anaesthesiologist. Three types of indicators (monitors); physical, chemical and biological are generally used in most hospitals to assess the efficiency of autoclaving or ethylene oxide sterilization. Some of these indicators which help in monitoring the efficiency of sterilization are also displayed in this section to remind the anaesthesiology residents that this aspect is also a matter of concern to them.

Chemical indicators change colour when certain conditions necessary for sterilization have been met. They are available as tapes, strips, cards and sheets. They may be implanted or attached to packaging material or enclosed in packages. Biological indicators give a greater surety of the proper functioning of any sterilizer and should be placed in the most inaccessible location in the sterilized load and then cultured. The only disadvantage of biological indicators is that they take several days to give results. While on this section it would be worthwhile mentioning the common disinfecting agents being utilized in our set up. Relevant literature on Cidex and Savlon are displayed. The technique of cold sterilization of the commonly used anaesthetic apparatus, respiratory therapy equipment, pressure transducers etc are mentioned in the appropriate heads. The method of surface and atmospheric, terminal and continuous disinfection by formaldehyde in operation suites and intensive care cubicles can efficiently be performed by aerosol disinfectors. A automist aerosol disinfector manufactured by Hatchwell Incubators, Hyderabad and being used in the Armed Forces hospitals has facilities for terminal neutralization of residual formalin by 25% ammonium hydroxide.

CARDIAC ANAESTHESIA

This aspect of anaesthesia continues to advance at a rapid pace. Many of the recent innovations in monitoring and pharmacology relevant to anaesthesiology had originated in the cardiac surgery theatres and then had wide application to patients with cardiac disease undergoing all types of surgery.

The most important and significant development in this sub specialty of anaesthesia was the invention of the "heart-lung machine" by John Gibbon and its first use in man in May 1953 and subsequently modified by Kirklin at the Mayo Clinic in 1957 as the Gibbon-Mayo stationary screen oxygenator. The success of cardiopulmonary by pass (CPB) is however equally owed to Howell's accidental discovery of Heparin; the principal anticoagulant in use today.

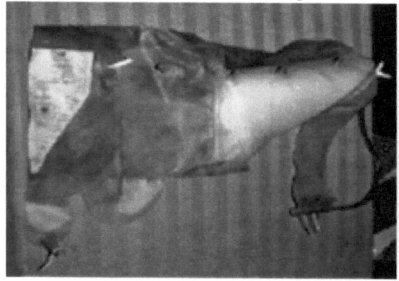 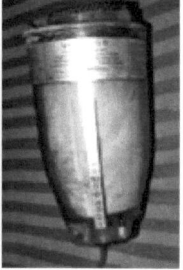

Oxygenators were the next item to be developed. Initial screen oxygenators that were followed by rotating disc oxygenators; but were soon superseded by the bubble oxygenators eg. **Rygg-Kysgaard** from Denmark and the **Spiraflo Bosio** of Bentley lab. The main criticism of these oxygenators was the presence of a blood-gas interface which leads to denaturation of plasma proteins and subsequent complications. This necessitated cutting down on the bypass time. The primary complications of operations requiring CPB are neurological abnormalities, renal failure, and post-operative respiratory insufficiency "pump-lung".

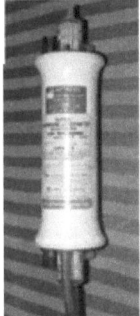

Membrane oxygenators (e.g., Sci Med of Life Systems Inc) which employ a silicone rubber membrane overcomes this difficulty but recent studies on advantages of such oxygenators which are extremely expensive has been questioned. Stress now is being laid on other parameters such as flow rates, perfusion pressures, haematocrit, filtration and temperature; accordingly, protocols for perfusion standards vary from center to center.

Nevertheless, mortality and morbidity due to cardiopulmonary bypass (CPB) is approaching lower values ever than before. Of interest now in the last decade of the 20th century has been the refinement and development of apparatus for CPB for the purpose of neonatal paediatric cardiac surgery. Nowadays the venous reservoir, oxygenator and heat exchanger with filter are incorporated as a single unit. As would be appropriate in this section are displayed models depicting the common cardiac lesions namely Atrial septal defect, PDA, Aberrant right subclavian artery, Tricuspid stenosis/insufficiency, Mitral stenosis/insufficiency and atrial stenosis. The importance and recognition of these lesions by any practicing anaesthesiologist is the obvious message that these models convey. Charts depicting the normal intracardiac pressures and oxygen saturation are displayed alongside in order to understand the physiological changes that accompany these pathological lesions.

The field of intensive care medicine is the most dynamic, volatile, diverse and creative than any other area in medicine. More and more countries all over the world are showing concern over the intensive care facilities in their communities and are widening the scope of progressive patient care of which intensive care is the foremost element. By virtue of the fact that anaesthesiologists have become experts in the principles of resuscitation and supportive care the onus of looking after critical care units has fallen on them. This by no means is a rule. On the contrary a new specialty is now in the offing and the doctors aspiring for such a specialty are being known as intensivists.

CRITICAL CARE

In this section the endeavor is not to define the structure design, working, advantages /disadvantages but the facilities that ought to be available in any set up. An ICU bed which can easily be maneuvered to suit various postures of the patient; have attachments for a feeding table, I/V infusion stand; facility for removal of back rest to help in case of intubation; a CPR board for effective cardiac compression; facility for sliding an X- ray film; railings attachment for restless or convulsing patients; and castors for transporting the patient on bed itself, is the most important item around which all other ancillaries can be revolve. Though providing an air current mattress on such beds is a dream, the Alfa/Betabed-Huntleigh Technology, and Mouslo Foam mattress- Europe Medical useful and cheaper devices that can be helpful for nursing comatose patients requiring frequent change of posture for prevention of bed sores.

The recommended space area of a cubicle for a single bed is 18 M^2. The next most important items in an ICU cubicle are the central pipe line outlets for O_2, N_2O, air and suction units (e.g. IOL vacuum units) with their attachments and ancillaries (suction catheters). A suction catheter device for use without disconnecting the patient from the ventilator (mfd. by Portex) is exhibited. Next in priority would be the infusion and transfusion pumps (e.g. Diginfusa, Lamtec pressure infusion box). Patient controlled analgesia (PCA) devices are increasingly being utilized by doctors who care for pain relief. All patients admitted to the ICU have three factors (need for ventilatory support, need for cardiovascular support, need for intense monitoring) in common. Any of the three may be required simultaneously or individually. Mortality and morbidity in anaesthesia are also attributed to the withdrawal of the intense intraoperative monitoring in the post-operative period. Hence all the monitoring especially that was defined in the minimum monitoring standards ought to be continued in the post-operative course for at least 48 hours. In the ICU's the trend is to have a bed side monitoring system which is connected to a central station where a single person can simultaneously monitor all the patients in the ICU. Very sophisticated computerized monitoring systems (e.g. PCMS/4-Spacelabs, Horizon 2200) whose cost is no doubt prohibitive are available. Up to 40 parameters actual and calculated can be displayed simultaneously in these monitors. They have additional facilities to float data from one bedside monitor to the other, detect abnormal rhythms and ischaemic patterns with their interpretation, store the data in memory which can be recalled later at any time and display the changing trends.

There are other support equipment which may not be able to be provided in each bed cubicle but are required to be ready near the central station for as and when required basis. These include the Crash Cart (Emergency drug trolley, Intubation drill equipment, Manual resuscitators, Emergency tracheotome, Central Venous and Pulmonary artery catheters), Monitor cum Defibrillator. A Portable Stat Laboratory (ABG analyser, Serum electrolytes, Sugar and NPN), A micro-processor ventilator with various ventilatory modes, Renal failure emergency kit (e.g. Gambro), Image Intensifier for cardiac pacing, Portable X-ray machine and Cardiac support devices (External and internal pacemakers, Intra-aortic balloon pump, Heart lung machine) are more sophisticated equipment necessary in a modern ICU. Other equipment that could be listed and that have a therapeutic value are fibre optic bronchoscope, fibre optic gastroscope, oxygen therapy appliances including hyperbaric oxygen chamber.

CONCLUSION

A comprehensive account of all what is available in this museum is discussed in this manuscript. Additional information on the subject is added at places to give more coverage on the topic and guide a resident on some aspects he or she may have missed during study. A number of books, journals and reviews have been consulted to give authenticity to this manuscript. It is hoped that it will not only serve as a guide to whoever visits the museum but also to give an idea to the under graduate students as to the amount of knowledge that is required to be acquired in the specialty of Anaesthesiology.

The talents desired of a safe anaesthetist are aptitude of a physician, academic ability, enthusiasm and energy, humanity, team membership concept, mental stability, sense of humour and conscientiousness. The International Society on preventable mortality and morbidity (ISPMM) in 1984 has outlined the unfit qualities of an anaesthetist. If one is absent minded, arrogant, careless, deceitful, disorderly, forgetful, headstrong, irresponsible, lazy, obnoxious and quarrelsome he must be discouraged from joining the specialty. The medical fraternity and the public at large require the services of not only a learned anaesthesiologist but more important a safe anaesthesiologist. To make a safe anaesthesiologist should be the role of any teacher in this important specialty of medicine.

REFERENCES

1. Adams A.P., (1992). Safety in anaesthetic practice in Recent Advances in Anaesthesia and
Analgesia No.17.
2. Breslow M.J., Miller C.F., Rogers M., (1990). Perioperative management. The C.V.Mosby
Company. St. Louis, Missouri.
3. Bruce W.,(1990). Anaesthetic Breathing Systems. In The scientific foundations of
anaesthesia the basis of intensive care. Fourth Ed.(Cyril Scurr, Stanley Feldman, Neil Soni)
Heinemann Medical Books, Oxford.
4. Calverley R.K.,(1992). Anaesthesia as a speciality: Past, present and future in Introduction to anaesthetic practice.
5. Davison M.H.A.,(1965). The evolution of anaesthesia. John Sherratt and Son, Altrincham.
6. Dorsch J.A., Dorsch S.E.,(1984). Understanding anaesthesia equipment.
Construction, care and complications. Second Ed. Williams & Wilkins. Baltimore/London.
7. Lee A.J., Atkinson R.S.,(1964). A synopsis of anaesthesia. Fifth Ed. John Wright and Sons Ltd. Bristol.
8. McLanthan, Richard,(1981). The directory of world museums. Second Ed.In New Standard
Encyclopaedia, Vol 11. Standard EducationalCorporation. Chicago.
9. Minnitt R.J., Gillies J.,(1945). Textbook of anaesthetics. Sixth Ed. E. & S. Livingstone Ltd.,
Teviot Place, Edinburgh.

10. Mushin W.W., Jones P.L.,(1987). Physics for the anaesthetist. Fourth Ed. Blackwell Scientific Publications. Oxford/London.

11. Pramanik S.,(1980). History of evolution of anaesthesia in India. Ind. J. Anaesth.,28,95.

12. Rama Rao, Khandekar S.N., (1960). Evolution of anaesthesia in the Armed Forces.Ind J. Anaesth., 8,99.

13. Stoelting K.J., Miller R.D.,(1984). Basics of anaesthesia. Churchill Livingstone Inc. New York.

14. Sykes W.S., (1960). Essays on the first hundred years of anaesthesia. Vol 1. E. & S. Livingstone Ltd., Teviot Place, Edinburgh.

15. Thornton H.L., Norton-Perkins H.D.,(1974). Emergency anaesthesia. Second Ed. Edward Arnold Ltd. London.

16. Ward C.S.,(1975). Anaesthetic equipment, Physical principles and Maintenance. Bailliere Tindall, London.

17. Wylie W.D., Churchill-Davidson H.C.,(1972). A practice of anaesthesia. Lloyd-Luke (Medical Books) Ltd. London.

www.ingramcontent.com/pod-product-compliance
Lightning Source LLC
Chambersburg PA
CBHW040223220526
45473CB00001B/93